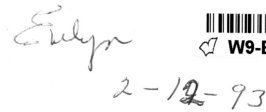

W9-BCO-609

THE LAZY PERSON'S GUIDE

TO BETTER NUTRITION

By Gordon S. Tessler, Ph.D.

Illustrator: Pamela Beets
Cover Photography: ReGina L. Raasch

For more information contact:

Dr. Gordon S. Tessler
c/o The Genesis Way
809 Spring Forest Road, Suite 1200
Raleigh, N.C.   27609
919-790-8888

Printed in the United States

DEDICATION

To my Creator, the God of Abraham, Isaac and Jacob, who is the author and finisher of my faith; to my parents, Jack and Erna.

ACKNOWLEDGEMENT

I thank God Almighty for His everlasting love and mercy. He has made this book possible.

ABOUT THE AUTHOR

Gordon S. Tessler, Ph.D., is a nationally recognized nutrition consultant, teacher, lecturer, and accomplished author. he is a personal student of the late Dr. Paavo Airola, world renown nutritionist, naturopathic physician, award-winning author, founder and past president of the International Academy of Biological Medicine. His studies have taken him to France, Germany, England, Spain, Sweden, Great Britain, and India. His extensive lecture schedule includes church groups, law enforcement agencies, medical groups, faculty and students of public schools, as well as the general public. His comprehensive seminars on Nutrition and Biblical Health are in great demand.

Dr. Tessler advocates nutritional therapy in the rehabilitation of drug abuse, alcoholism, eating disorders, smoking withdrawal, depression, emotional instability, and other such problems aggravated by chemical imbalances in the body, as well as reducing degenerative diseases such as heart disease, cancer, diabetes and arthritis in the general population. He believes that a wellness lifestyle, including nutrition and exercise, will maintain optimum health throughout a person's life.

TABLE OF CONTENTS

INTRODUCTION

"ASK NOT WHAT YOUR BODY CAN DO FOR YOU: ASK WHAT YOU CAN DO FOR YOUR BODY!"

THE LAZY PERSON'S GUIDE TO BETTER NUTRITION is a manual to guide and help you understand what **you** can do for your body. Your body is just like you; it needs **love** and attention! When you love someone you place value in them — you give them your time, energy, attention and money. Similarly, practicing better nutrition is a form of love. In order to be a healthy person, you must develop a positive and dynamic relationship with your body, learning to listen to it, care for it and value it. After all, since you are only given one body for your stay on earth, the two of you might as well become friends!

The nutritional field is packed with information and **misinformation** adding stress and confusion to our already over-complicated lives. Most people's problem regarding nutrition is not a lack of belief, but rather, believing everything. Although most people agree that nutrition is important for maintaining good health, many nutritionists disagree on the best diet to follow.

The work of two pioneer nutritionists, Drs. Paavo Airola and Bernard Jensen, offer a path out of this nutrition jungle. Their separately conducted studies of the living and eating habits of cultures known for superior health and longevity give clues to a lifestyle that has worked for generations. Therefore these concepts **can work for you!!**

Several examples of such healthy cultures include the Hunzhuts of Pakistan, the Abkhazaians of Russia, the Bulgarians, the traditional Japanese, the Vilcabambas of Equador and the Yucatan and the Chihuahua Indians of Mexico. These cultures have unique, but easily attainable eating habits. In **THE LAZY PERSON'S GUIDE TO BETTER NUTRITION,** you will learn the lifestyle maintained for centuries by these cultures, resulting in long and fruitful lives.

i

Your health is the most valuable possession you have. With good health, you can do anything. Without it, you couldn't earn money, support your family or love and enjoy life. Everything would be a tremendous struggle without your health. I know people who have spent all their energies acquiring the comforts of life . . .cars, homes, power, prestige, family, etc., only to find they have lost their health in the climb to the top. Such people would gladly exchange all their possessions for a few more weeks of life.

What you eat is not harmless; what you eat either helps or hurts! Some people have been misguided into believing that what they eat has little relationship to their health. **WRONG!** Don't believe it! Your lifestyle today, including what you eat, determines your health for tomorrow, and year after year. **Although practicing intelligent nutrition may not add years to your life, it will add life to your years.**

Your lifestyle has more to do with your health than anything else. The bad news is that we create our own sickness. The good news, put forth in this guide, is that YOU can create your own good health. By avoiding the Standard American Diet (S.A.D.) which causes much unnecessary suffering, and by adopting the lifestyle of cultures renowned for their good health, YOU will provide yourself with a nutritional bank account which can handle anything life sends your way!

Maybe what you don't know can't hurt you, but more importantly, what you don't know certainly won't help you. When you develop an awareness of nutrition and daily wholesome eating, nutritious foods act like a savings account. By putting money in a savings account regularly, you prepare yourself for a financial emergency If you do not save regularly, you may need a loan when a crisis strikes. Consequently, as financial pressures continue, more borrowing follows until possible bankruptcy results. Similarly, optimum nutrition acts as a savings account which assures and insures that the stresses of modern living can be met. If you do not eat well, take supplements and exercise regularly, your body borrows calcium and magnesium from your bones and teeth, B-Complex from your nervous system, Vitamin A from your cell membranes, and has NO intention of repaying the debt.

Vitamin and mineral deficiencies are the beginnings of disease. **Disease is nutritional bankruptcy.**

The amount of time, money and suffering involved to regain lost health is certainly not the Lazy Person's way. Remember, a Lazy Person invented the wheel! To save time and money, the safest and most direct path is to practice the Lazy Person's motto: **"Maintaining health is easier than regaining health."**

The Lazy Person is **not** in a hurry. Along with the modern diseases of heart disease, cancer and diabetes, the **hurry disease** needs to be included. **If you are not in a hurry to live, you probably won't be in a hurry to die.** The Lazy Person travels at a safe speed through life, making the time to smell flowers, enjoy sunrises and sunsets and relish just being ALIVE! THE LAZY PERSON'S GUIDE TO BETTER NUTRITION teaches you to install your own brakes by listening to your body. When your blood pressure rises, you're going TOO fast!

THE LAZY PERSON'S GUIDE TO BETTER NUTRITION is for you whether you are a beginner or a weekend health nut. **Nutrition is not a fad, but rather a matter of life and death.** If you want to cash in on the interest from a Nutritional Savings Account . . .eating better, feeling better, being healthier and happier. . . this book will be your informative, enjoyable and inspirational guide. Have fun!

Gordon S. Tessler, Ph.D.

AUTHOR'S PREFACE

I find health and the pursuit of health is more infectious than disease. As you improve your lifestyle, a richer way of life becomes possible.

The earth's history is filled with accounts of golden opportunities that people have had and ignored. Such a golden opportunity is now available to you. As you well know, a Lazy Person is not afraid of hard work, only of wasting time going in the wrong direction.

Moving in the direction of wellness offers you less pain, greater highs and fewer lows. You will congratulate yourself in a year or so for having begun a new, healthier lifestyle. The majority of failures in the world are not those who try and do not succeed, but those who are afraid to start. **It does not matter where you are now standing, only in which direction you are moving.**

I would like to tell you how I began my love affair with nutrition. Many of my fellow practitioners were chronically ill at one time in their lives, and I was no exception. I was a sickly child, with countless strep throats, colds, impetigo, and finally at the age of twelve, I contracted an "incurable" skin disease called Psoriasis.

Psoriasis is an ugly and embarressing condition, especially to a young teenager. I wore long-sleeved shirts and turtlenecks, combed my hair in bangs (before the Beatles made this style popular) . . .anything to cover up the red, scaly patches that itched constantly. During the early treatment of this condition, the doctor's only recourse was to rub the scales off with alcohol while I screamed. **I felt like I had leprosy!** I became shy, withdrawn and lacked confidence throughout my high school years. I never dated, because I thought no girl would go out with me. My dermatologist, who did all he thought he could do for me, told me Psoriasis was "incurable." The medication and x-ray treatments I took kept the sores manageable, but if I ever missed an appointment with the doctor, I would have another flair-up.

When I was almost eighteen, I read a nutrition book that insisted Psoriasis was related to improper fat metabolism in the liver. The book suggested that the Psoriasis victim give up beef, pork and veal to improve the condition. I was desperate, so I stopped eating red meat. After six weeks on this program, 90% of my Psoriasis disappeared!! Meanwhile, I was still eating junk food of all kinds — the only change I had made in my life was to remove red meat from my diet. I told my dermatologist about my experiment. I vividly remember my doctor shaking his head as if to say, You are really misguided, Gordon. He told me, firmly, "There is no relationship between diet and disease."

Looking back on this incident, which happened twenty years ago, I realize I knew something that my doctor did not: **how you feel is related to what you eat.** When I learned this secret, I wanted to stop people on the streets and shout, "You don't have to be sick; nature heals!" Just as putting the correct fuel in an automobile allows the engine to run well, eating a nutritious diet of whole foods allows our bodies to be full of energy to meet the challenges of living.

The tendency to want to tell the world about health is very natural. When beginning any new program, we have great enthusiasm without much actual experience. We are like a match flame; any slight wind can easily blow it out. However, after practicing nutrition for several months, our flame transforms into a great bonfire which not even a hurricane can extinguish.

The Lazy Person's way (for those of us who want to succeed with the least amount of pain and suffering) is to keep our truth to ourselves until even non-support or negativity will not extinguish our well established flame of experience. **The best sermon is preached by your actions and not by your lips.** When a rose blooms, it doesn't have to call the bees, animals or humans; its beauty and fragrance will attract sufficient attention. As you begin to radiate new found energy and health, people will be drawn to you. When your friends or co-workers say, "Gee, you look great!" or "Haven't you lost weight?", this will be the time to proclaim the power of your new nutritional habits and lifestyle. The flame of your healthier lifestyle will become the example, lighting the way for others. **Live your life well, because you may be the only nutrition book someone ever reads.** There are few people who can succeed in a new endeavor without some outside support. May I suggest that you choose your support very carefully. As you become healthier, you may experience criticism from those you felt would be happy for you. You will be changing your life and taking a risk that many others do not have the courage to consider. **Make it easy on yourself; keep quiet around those people who don't support you.** In days past, the saying was "don't throw your pearls before swine." If you are doing something that is important to you, share it with someone who cares, not with someone who will drain your energy. How much enthusiasm would a team have if the fans booed each score?

Read books on the subject of health and nutrition (see appendix). Go to lectures. Begin to study and respect your body; look at it for what it is: a marvelous and unique creation. My grandfather once said, **"If you take care of your body, your body will take care of you."** Your body is a walking miracle, equipped to mend damaged tissue, regenerate dying cells and eliminate waste products. Your body is a "faithful servant," regulating itself by maintaining such functions as body temperature, heart and respiratory rates, blood flow, blood pressure and acid-alkaline balance. As wonderful as it may be, your body cannot survive the punishment of **disuse, misuse and abuse** over many years.

THE LAZY PERSON'S GUIDE TO BETTER NUTRITION provides you with the knowledge needed to build optimum health. There is no end to how healthy you can be. Responsibility for your own health can help you avoid the high cost of medical care. Even God cannot steer a parked car. So start developing your new lifestyle today! Drive in the direction of health and use The Lazy Person's Guide as your map!

CHAPTER 1

THE OPTIMUM DIET FOR OPTIMUM HEALTH

"THE DOCTOR OF THE FUTURE WILL GIVE NO MEDICINE BUT WILL INTEREST HIS PATIENT IN THE CARE OF THE HUMAN FRAME, IN DIET, AND IN THE CAUSE AND PREVEN-TION OF DISEASE." Thomas A. Edison

Most nutritionists promote their own personal dietary ideas, causing confusion and contradiction in the nutritional field. **Studying dietary patterns that have enabled cultures to remain healthy and disease-free for generations is the only sensible and scientific means to determine the healthiest way to eat.** Most of the confusion and misinformation in nutritional literature would end if more nutritionists followed the examples of Dr. Paavo Airola and Dr. Bernard Jensen. Both of these doctors traveled worldwide studying cultures renowned for their superior health and longevity. Such extraordinary cultures include the traditional Japanese, the Equadorian Vikabambas, the Pakastanian Hunzahuts, the Bulgarians, the Yucatans and Chihuahua Indians of Mexico and the Abkhazians of Russia.

The United States, along with may other nations, was founded on the principles and precepts of other lands and peoples. Even the English language is a composite of Latin, Greek and German. Great Britian's traditions provided many of the ideas necessary for the formation of the original 13 colonies. The Olympic games of today are modeled after those in ancient Greece. Tradition, as defined in Webster's Dictionary, is "the handing down of beliefs and customs by word of mouth or example." If something works, and has worked for centuries, why not use it?

Healthy cultures of today have long and successful track records. Their civilizations exemplify lives free from heart

1

disease, cancer, diabetes and arthritis prevalent in many Americans. Although modern medicine and technology has practically eliminated contagious diseases plaguing the world for centuries, these diseases have been replaced with degenerative ones. A degenerative disease is **not** contagious; a person does not "catch" heart disease, cancer or diabetes, he develops the condition over time, a condition directly related to his/her lifestyle.

Healthy cultures have developed a lifestyle permitting full, energetic lives and natural deaths. One night, my grandfather went to bed as usual and did not wake up. That is considered a natural death, something which few Americans experience anymore. Instead, most die a premature death which is usually slow, painful and full of great suffering for themselves and their loved ones. Many nutritionists insist, **"Man doesn't die, he kills himself with his teeth."**

The time has come to take a Lazy Person's look at lifestyles of those cultures renown for superior health and longevity. Although scattered throughout the world, these cultures have strikingly similar eating and living habits. The following guidelines are not one nutritionist's opinion of what you should eat; rather they provide a "health map" which has kept people well for generations. This formula indicates the most eaten foods, the least eaten foods and the percentage of each food commonly found in the world's healthiest people. Since this diet has kept people healthy for generations, the formula is called **"The Optimum Diet for Optimum Health."**

OPTIMUM DIET FOR OPTIMUM HEALTH

Food	% IN DIET
1. Grains, Beans, Seeds, Nuts	50%
2. Vegetables	30%
3. Fruits	10%
4. Dairy Products	6%
5. Meat (fish, fowl, beef, pork, lamb)	4%

Food Group	% IN DIET
1. Complex Carbohydrates	70-75%
2. Fats	15-20%
3. Protein	10%

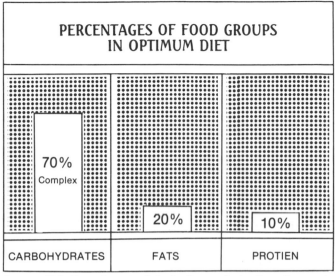

PERCENTAGES OF FOOD GROUPS IN OPTIMUM DIET

CARBOHYDRATES	FATS	PROTIEN
70% Complex	20%	10%

Source: U.S. Department of Agriculture - Agriculture Research Service.

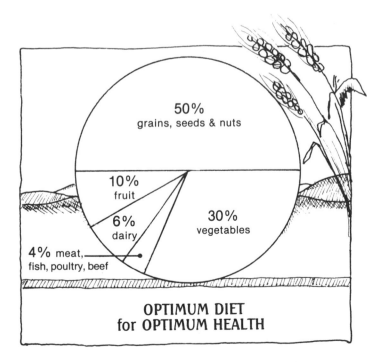

50%
grains, seeds & nuts

10%
fruit

6%
dairy

4% meat,
fish, poultry, beef

30%
vegetables

OPTIMUM DIET for OPTIMUM HEALTH

GRAINS

Airola's and Jensen's studies of healthy cultures outline the diet for superior health and disease prevention. **Grains, seeds and nuts are the staple foods which are eaten in greater percentages than any other (50%).** This food group is the most important, as it contains the nutrients necessary to maintain what Dr. Airola called "Optimum Health." Grains, beans, seeds and nuts such as buckwheat, pinto beans, lentils, millet, brown rice, pumpkin seeds, sesame seeds, sunflower seeds and almonds contain good quality protein (see Chapter Four). Grains are the best source of glucose, providing the healthy energy our bodies need. (see Chapter Three). Grains, seeds and nuts also have high levels of Vitamin A, E and B Complex along with nutritious amounts of most minerals and trace minerals.

The Hunzakut's staple grain is millet, the Japanese eat brown rice, the Yucatan and Chihuahua Indians eat corn and beans and the Abkhazian of Russia eat millet and buckwheat. After reading the Carbohydrates Chapter, you will understand why these concentrated and perfect foods became the staples of healthy cultures everywhere.

Most Americans believe that eating whole grain bread is the same as eating whole grains. When grain is milled into flour, decay begins rapidly, oxidizing vitamins and minerals. The remainder of nutrients not oxidized will be damaged when the flour is placed in the oven at 450 degrees for 45 minutes. The healthy cultures previously mentioned eat no bread. Instead, some of these cultures grind their own grain, add water and a pinch of salt, flatten the mixture into a pancake and brown it on both sides, resulting in a corn or wheat tortilla. These cultures do not add milk, oil, eggs, sugar, honey, yeast or baking powder to their tortillas.

Our "spongy" bread, including most whole grain bread, tends to absorb water within our bodies which congests the small and large intestines. This congestion results in constipation. Whole grains, on the other hand, are high fiber foods which improve elimination.

Grains, are composed of phytic acid or phytates. Phytic acid, found in the outer part of the kernal, maintains the

4

molecular bonding necessary to prevent grains from decay. **If phytates are not broken down by sprouting or cooking, some minerals, especially calcium, will be depleted from the body.** Rice and millet are the lowest in phytic acid. Grains may be cooked in water, at a low heat or baked in an oven. Rolled oats are already cooked by the heat produced in the rolling process.

NUTS AND SEEDS

Nuts and seeds when eaten raw and unsalted, contain complete protein, minerals and trace minerals, and have more pantothenic acid (needed to fight stress) than any other food except liver. Raw nuts and seeds are also rich in the fertility vitamin, Vitamin E and supply large amounts of calcium and zinc.

Nuts and seeds should never be heated or roasted, as this procedure causes their important unsaturated fats to become rancid. Remember that rancid oil can produce free radicals in your body which can cause cancer.

VEGETABLES

Vegetables constitute the second food group (30%), and are excellent sources of vitamins and minerals. Potatoes, squash, cabbage, carrots and greens provide fiber and glucose for optimum energy. The proteins contained in alfalfa and leaf vegetables are comparable to the protein found in cow's milk. Vegetables may be baked, steamed or eaten raw in salad form.

FRUITS

Fruits are catagorized as the third most important food group (10%). Like vegetables, fruits are excellent sources of vitamins and minerals. They are easily digested sugars and have a wonderful cleansing effect on the bloodstream and digestive tract. Although fruit takes approximately 80 minutes to reach the bloodstream (preferable to the eight seconds refined sugar takes), too much fruit will upset the sugar balance. **Eating a few almonds with fruit, and eliminating dried fruit for those of you who have severe hypoglycemia, will protect individuals from unpleasant side**

effects of low blood sugar. As most commercial fruit is picked green, sugars do not properly mature, and fruit acid content is high. Therefore, gas, bloating and diarrhea result when fruit is overconsumed. I recommend two whole fruits a day in the winter and, more in the summer when the cooling effect of raw, fresh fruit is especially important. As with vegetables, eat fruit according to the season.

The three food groups previously mentioned: grains, seeds and nuts, vegetables and fruits, constitute the majority (90%) of all foods eaten by healthy cultures who have great endurance, sound teeth, little or no degenerative diseases, work up to 16 hours a day and live a long, energetic life — some as long as 100 years!

DAIRY

Few dairy products (6%) are consumed in cultures known for extraordinary health. The milk products used are cultured such as yogurt, kefir, cottage cheese and butter-milk. I recommend no dairy products for people of Japanese, Chinese or African descent (see Chapter Nine), and up to **four ounces of yogurt or other cultured milk products** a day for people of European descent.

MEAT

If you wish to eat from the fifth food group (4%), **fish is your best alternative.** Fish contains no artificial hormones or antibiotics. Shell fish such as shrimp, lobster, clams, scallops and crab are not recommended. Shell fish are scavengers who eat all the "junk" in the ocean. They are the garbage collectors of the sea, just as rats, flies and buzzards are on land, and may be termed the "rats of the ocean." Skin fish such as shark, cat fish, turbo and carp are almost as unclean as shellfish. Additionally, due to its high levels of mercury, tuna is also not recommended.

Fish may be prepared by boiling, baking or poaching. Many healthy cultures eat a little fish, utilizing its high phosphorus content (brain food) along with Vitamins A and D. This diet is an excellent alternative to heavier proteins such as poultry and meat. Buy fish fresh or frozen from your local supermarket, health food store or fresh fish market.

Chicken and turkey are preferred alternatives to beef, pork and veal since they contain lower levels of fat and chemical additives.

When purchasing poultry or beef, find distributors that sell products which were raised naturally. Corn fed animals with no hormone or antibiotic additives taste far superior and are much healthier for you than their commercial counterparts. Reduce your meat consumption to 2 or 3 times a week, and eat mainly fish. Remember that healthy cultures eat meat sparingly, usually once a month. A reduction in consumption of this food group poses no health threats and **will** reduce the unneeded fat and cholesterol (see Chapter Four).

The Standard American Diet (S.A.D.) is exactly opposite the "Optimum Diet for Optimum Health" plan. The S.A.D. has a very poor track record, as high rates of heart disease, diabetes and cancer indicate.

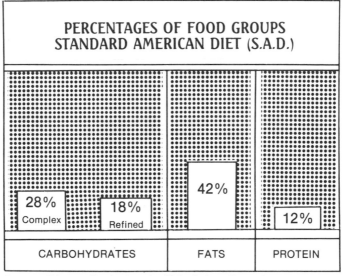

Source: Dietary Goals for the U.S. Select Committee on Nutritional & Human Needs U.S. Senate.

Our carbohydrate consumption from starches such as potatoes and whole grains have been cut back by 45% since 1910. However, consumption of refined carbohydrates has increased by 31%, while fat consumption has increased 28% (56% increase in fats from butter, margerine, oil, etc.) since 1910.

CHANGES IN NUTRIENT CONSUMPTION Per Capita for U.S. 1910 – 1976		
CALORIES	1910-76	−3%
FAT	1910-76	+ 28%
CARBOHYDRATES	1910-76	−21%
PROTEIN	1910-76	+ 1%
DIETARY FAT from separated fats (butter, margarine, oil etc.)	1921-76	+ 56%
CARBOHYDRATES Grams (from sugars)	1909-13— 1976	+ 31%
CARBOHYDRATES Grams (from starches)	1909-13— 1976	−45%

Source: *Changing American Diet* by the Center for Science in the Public Interest.

WHAT TO EAT

Grains   Brown rice, rolled oats (no Quick Oats), millet, buckwheat, barley, rye, corn meal and wheat berries. Soy is not recommended unless of Oriental descent. The trypsin inhibitors (enzyme for proteins) in soy make it indigestible to westerners.

Beans and Legumes	Pinto, black (turtle, not soy) garbanzo, azuki, black-eyed peas, lentils, lima, kidney, split peas. To make beans "less musical," soak in water for 24 hours, pour off water and cook. Cooking with kelp or other sea vegetables helps.
Nuts	Almonds are the king of nuts and the only alkaline nut. Other nuts that are nutritious, although acid forming, are pecans, filberts, walnuts, brazil nuts and pinon. **Peanuts, high in fat, are almost indigestable to humans.** For best digestion of cashews and peanuts, cook in soups only.
Seeds	Sunflower, pumpkin, sesame, flax, chia, psyllium.
Vegetables	Potatoes (red, sweet, and yams have more protein and Vitamin C than Irish), carrots, cauliflower, artichokes, asparagus, squash (yellow, zuccini, acorn, hubbard, spaghetti), green beans, tomatoes, beets and beet greens, broccoli, brussel sprouts, red and green cabbage, Chinese cabbage, celery, collards, corn, cucumber, endive, kale, Jerusalem artichokes, mushrooms, leeks, onions, lettuce (romaine, bibb, red leaf), kohlrabi, okra, parsley, green pepper, parsnips, peas, pumpkin, turnips, watercress (to name a few).
Fruits	Apples (all varieties), pears, apricots, peaches, avocados, bananas, blackberries, raspberries, blueberries, strawberries, cherries, cantaloupe, casaba melon, watermelon, cranberries, currants, dates, raisins, figs, grapefruit, oranges, honeydew melon, mangos, papayas, persimmons, pineapple, plums, pomegranate, prunes, tangerines and rhubarb.

Herbs and Spices	Garlic, ginger root, onions, parsley, basil, sage, tumeric, curry, bay leaf, cardamon, chili powder, coriander, cumin, dill, fennel, marjoram, mustard seed, oregano, paprika, cayenne, cinnamon, nutmeg, rosemary, saffron, tarragon.
Fish	Bass, cod, flounder, haddock, halibut, perch, pike, sole, salmon, red snapper, trout. Any other **scaled** fresh water or ocean fish is acceptable.
Meat	Beef, lamb, chicken and turkey (should be free of hormones, chemicals and antibiotics). Call a health food store for information on where to find these particular products. Whole grain casseroles are a good meat dish replacement.
Sea Vegetables	Agar-agar, dulse, kelp, kombu and nori.

Cooking

Every cell eats, digests and eliminates food just as we do. The wonderful life in food is the same life we have within us. What would happen to your life if I threw you in boiling oil, boiling water or in a 450 degree oven, just as many of us do with our food? Your body chemistry would undergo a deadly change. On the other hand, if I placed you in a sauna or steam bath for a few minutes, would you survive? Of course! Nutritionists recommend steaming your food so its nutritional value is maintained. **Steaming, cooking or baking foods at low heat maintains nutritional value.**

WHEN TO EAT
"Life is more digestive if it is sipped, not gulped."

Americans tend to be gluttons when they eat. This unhealthy habit may be attributed to waiting three to five hours or longer between meals. Such waiting depletes the blood sugar, leaving a person tired and famished. By the time we do eat, our blood sugar is so low we tend to over eat and never feel full. Gluttony is a harmful practice, as the "stuffing" of food only serves to overwork the digestive system. Food is digested and absorbed very poorly when such eating habits are followed, tending to encourage fat storage.

"Grazing" describes the eating patterns of healthy cultures. **Eating several small meals a day is the healthiest practice one can follow.** Several small snacks a day (four to six) stabilizes blood sugar without overworking or overfilling the stomach. In its healthy and mature state, the stomach is about the size of a fist. It only needs a small amount of food to be satisfied. This can be accomplished by frequent, small meals.

Have you ever noticed the way small children and babies eat? They are satisfied with several small meals a day. They will eat half a banana, run outside to play, come back in an hour for a little cheese then run back outside again. Children prefer snacking throughout the day. However, parents are taught eating between meals spoils a child's appetite. Therefore, they starve their children for several hours and then expect them to eat a large meal like "grown-ups." **The three-meal-a-day habit makes gluttons out of children who are natural "grazers."**

Many of my clients ask me if eating so many small meals overworks the digestive organs. The answer is no, but too much food at one meal does. Does breathing over and over again hurt the lungs? If it did, a person would have to take one gigantic breath and hold it in for three hours! It is natural to put food in the digestive tract. **And frequent, small meals will discourage over-eating and gluttony.**

Small meals help you lose weight, keeping those unwanted pounds off permanently! A study involving two groups of people at a major university proved that **how you eat is just as important as what you eat.** Both groups were given two thousand calories of food a day. Both group's foods were identical. However, one group was given eight meals a day of two hundred fifty calories per meal, the other group was given two meals of one thousand calories per meal. **The group eating two large meals a day gained weight, while the group who was allowed frequent, small meals lost weight!**

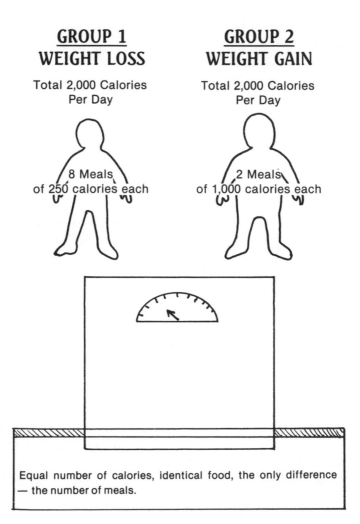

GROUP 1
WEIGHT LOSS

Total 2,000 Calories
Per Day

8 Meals
of 250 calories each

GROUP 2
WEIGHT GAIN

Total 2,000 Calories
Per Day

2 Meals
of 1,000 calories each

Equal number of calories, identical food, the only difference
— the number of meals.

Since our bodies utilize approximately two hundred and fifty calories per hour during normal activity, all these calories would be burned up if only that amount were consumed. On the other hand, calories consumed above and beyond the normal requirement of two hundred and fifty would be stored as fat.

A small amount of food is easily digested, while large amounts of food turn our stomachs into garbage cans. The examples of children and healthy cultures remind us that frequent, small meals keep our energy levels stable and never overburden our stomachs.

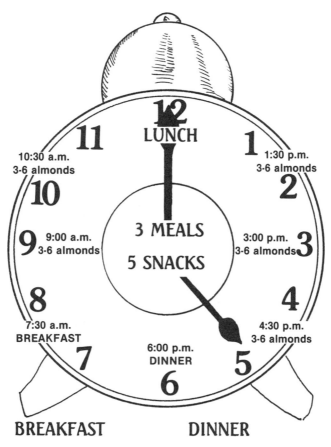

BREAKFAST   DINNER

Times are approximate. Tailor your own eating schedule. It is important to eat snacks 1½ hours apart to maintain stable blood sugar level.

Breakfast

This meal needs to consist of grains such as oats (see recipes) in order to keep our blood sugar stable until noon. Feeling full for a few hours after eating a grain meal is a sign that your blood sugar is stable.

Lunch

This meal varies according to circumstance and convenience. Many fast-food chains have salad bars, an excellent choice for lunch. Seek out natural food restaurants or cafeterias near your office, or bring your own lunch to work (see recipes).

Dinner

I suggest dinner be a family meal if possible. In the United States today, 50% of all food dollars are spent **outside the home** at fast-food chains. This unhealthy practice is expensive and contributes to the breakdown of marriages and families. **Bring your family together at dinner!** Grain should be eaten at this meal, if not already eaten at lunch. **For increased energy and elimination, grains have to be eaten at breakfast and again at lunch or dinner.**

Snacks

If energy is low, eat protein snacks such as almonds, sunflower seeds or yogurt. Fruits also are delicious snacks, but can upset blood sugar unless eaten with protein. A few almonds eaten with fruit will stabilize the blood sugar. **Do not wait longer than two hours between snacks.** Very light snacks may also be eaten in the evening if necessary. Restful sleep is assured if protein is not eaten too late at night, since protein takes at least eight hours to digest. **Make sure your stomach is asleep before you are.**

RECIPES

BREAKFAST SUGGESTIONS

Outstanding Oats (my clients' favorite breakfast)

1. Soak 1/2 cup rolled oats and 2 tbsp. currants in distilled water overnight.
    In the morning:
    Pour off water from oats and add:
    1   banana (sliced)
    1   tbsp. plain yogurt (optional)
    1   grated apple (optional)
    10 almonds (grind in blender) or whole
    Stir and enjoy.

For hot oatmeal:
    Pour boiling water over 1/2 cup rolled oats and currants, cover steep for 5 minutes. Pour off water and add above ingredients.

Multi-Grain Cereal

Use one or more:
Cracked wheat, millet, steel oats, barley, rye, buckwheat (for freshness, crack grains in blender as you use them).

1. Soak 1/3 cup multi-grain cereal in distilled water overnight.
   In the morning:
   Pour off the water and rinse again.
2. Soak separately overnight:
   1/4 cup unsweetened apple juice
   2 tbsp. raw almonds (whole)
   2 tbsp. currants
   1/4 teaspoon chia seeds

In the morning:
Place rinsed cereal and soaked apple juice mixture in blender. Blend until smooth. Enjoy.

Buckwheat Pancakes

1 cup buckwheat flour
1/3 cup rice flour or soy flour
2 eggs
1 cup buttermilk or yogurt, or kefir
If batter is too thick add water.

Mix buckwheat flour and rice flour, then add other ingredients. Use butter or sesame oil in pan, and use apple juice concentrate (Jensen) or apple sauce for a topping.

Corn Mush

Boil 1 cup water.
In a separate bowl, mix 1 cup cold water with 1 cup corn meal (course grain is best).
Add to boiling water ¼ cup of currants or raisins.
Simmer and stir occasionally for 5 to 7 minutes.
Add banana or other fresh fruit.
Use Apple Concentrate to sweeten (Jensen).

LUNCH AND DINNER SUGGESTIONS

If you're out to lunch . . .

If you're out to lunch,
as many people are,
then try a Salad Bar.
Add a potato or some fish,
and you'll have a very nice dish.

Wok Veggies and Rice

3 cups water
1 cup brown rice

Boil water, add rice (millet may be substituted), simmer for 45 minutes, or bake in oven at 350 degrees with 2 cups water, 1 cup brown rice. Fifteen minutes before rice is done, cook veggies in wok or saute in pan. (Use sesame oil or olive oil, and Quick Sip).

1 large carrot
1/2 leek or onion
2 small red potatoes
1/3 lb. of firm tofu or chicken (optional)
1 cup kale, broccoli or cauliflower.

Add cooked rice, and continue stirring 2 minutes over medium heat.

Mexican Fiesta Tostada

2 cups pinto beans
Soak overnight.
Boil for 4-5 hours (or until done). Add one large diced onion and 2 large cloves garlic (diced).
When beans are done, whip until smooth.
Put beans on corn tortilla.* Garnish with chopped lettuce and tomatoes. Add Mexican hot sauce and guacamole if desired.
*Bake tortilla for 5 minutes in oven or until crisp.

16

Mexican Hot Sauce

6 large tomatoes blended
2   8 oz. jars tomato sauce (salt free)
6 diced green chilies
2 diced jalapenos
1 large onion, diced
4 large cloves garlic, diced
1 tbsp. red chili powder
1 tbsp. ground cumin
1 tsp. ground oregano
2 cups water

Bring to a boil; simmer for 15 minutes. Yields 2 quarts.

Millet Delight (1 serving)

1 1/2 cup water
1/2 cup millet

Boil water; add millet; cover pot; simmer 20 minutes (check water and add as needed).
Millet should be fluffy, but not mushy or soggy.

Optional ingredients to add:
½ avocado (slice and mash into millet)
1 tbsp. olive oil
1 tomato
Quick Sip (Jensen)
Small amount of fresh lemon juice

Enjoy; this is an excellent, alkaline, easily digested meal, satisfying any protein or starch cravings.

Hummus

1½ cups uncooked or 3 cups cooked garbanzo beans
3 cloves garlic
1½ tsp. Vegit or Vegetable Broth (Jensen)
2 lemons
1/4 cup minced parsley
3/4 cup raw sesame tahini
1/4 tsp. cayenne pepper
1/3 tsp. cumin
2 tbsp. Quick Sip
1 cup liquid from cooked garbanzos

Cook garbanzo beans; peel garlic; wash and mince parsley. Put all but parsley and tahini in a blender and blend until smooth. Add remaining ingredients and hand mix until thoroughly combined. Cover and refrigerate til needed.   Yield: 3 cups

Use as a dip with unsalted corn chips or make a sandwich with lettuce and tomato.

CROCKPOT CAPERS

Your crockpot is an easy way to prepare delicious soups.

Mushroom Barley Soup

    1 lb. mushrooms, sliced
    2 cups barley (soak 12 hours before cooking)
    1 diced yellow onion
    Quick Sip and Vegetable Broth to taste
    2 cloves garlic
    Place ingredients in crockpot, fill crockpot with distilled or spring water and cook overnight on "low" setting.

Vegetable-Rice Potassium Soup

    1 sliced carrot
    2 sliced red potatoes
    1 yellow onion
    3 stalks diced celery
    diced parsley
    Quick Sip and Vegetable Broth to taste
    ½ cup brown rice
    chicken (optional)
    Place all ingredients in crockpot; fill crockpot with distilled or spring water, and cook overnight on "low" setting.

Lentil Potato Stew

    1 cup lentils
    3 red potatoes-chunks
    2 sliced carrots
    1 chopped yellow onion
    2 cloves chopped garlic
    2 stalks sliced celery
    Quick Sip and Vegetable Broth to taste
    Add water and cook overnight on "low" setting.

SALADS

Combination Vegetable Salad

Use 75% lettuce, celery, tomatoes, **plus 3 or 4 of the following:**

    Use all varieties of lettuce
    Carrots (tender and young)
    Beets and tops
    Cucumber
    Cauliflower
    Sweet peppers
    Fresh peas
    Bean sprouts
    Alfalfa sprouts
    Endive
    Escarole
    Swiss chard
    Chinese cabbage
    Jicama (hickima)
    Parsley
    Note: A little olive oil and lemon or other health dressing.

Tropical Fruit Salad

    2 ripe bananas
    1/2 medium pineapple
    2 ripe mangos
    1/2 pint blueberries or other berries
    1 papaya
    Cut up all ingredients, include juice, then add 1 cup finely
    ground almonds (grind in blender or nut grinder). Mix and
    enjoy!

SNACK IDEAS

Cuddley Carob Candy (for chocolate lovers)

    Melt 1 cup unsweetened carob chips in double boiler add
    2 tbsp. sesame butter
then add:
    1/2 lb. raw sunflower seeds
    1/2 lb. currants
    1/2 lb. sliced almonds
    2 tbsp. almond butter
    1/4 c almond milk*

Mix well, then spoon silver dollar size on cookie sheet and freeze for one-half hour.

*Add 6 almonds and ¼ c. water. Place in blender; blend until smooth.

Nut Mix (make your own)

1/2 lb. raw almonds
1/2 lb. sunflower seeds
1/2 lb. currants
1/2 lb. pumpkin seeds
1/2 lb. unsweetened shredded coconut

Mix together; and eat **only** a handful for a snack.

Yummie Yogurt

3 or 4 tbsp. of plain, unsweetened yogurt
1 banana and/or other fresh fruit
10 almonds or 2 tbsp. of sunflower seeds
2 tbsp. of Apple Concentrate (Jensen)

Mix together and enjoy between meals.

Apple Sauce

2 oz. unsweetened apple juice
1 diced apple
2 dates (pitted)

Blend together, place in bowl and add coconut and cinnamon.

CHAPTER 2

GUIDELINES FOR OPTIMUM HEALTH

"BE INTERESTED IN WHAT IS RIGHT, NOT WHO IS RIGHT."
Dr. Bernard Jensen

Eat Breakfast Please

Breakfast is considered by many nutrition experts to be the most important meal of the day. "Eat like a king at breakfast, like a queen at lunch and like a pauper at dinner," was an adage of a popular nutritionist. Many Americans eat little or no breakfast and indulge in a huge meal at dinner. If you eat a large and late dinner, you probably will not be hungry in the morning. And if you are one of those people who does not feel hungry in the morning, follow this simple rule: Never eat more at dinner than you ate at breakfast. If you didn't eat breakfast, don't eat dinner. I can guarantee that you will be hungry the next morning.

Eat In A Calm Environment

Eat in a calm and peaceful setting. **It is better not to eat when you are angry, nervous or otherwise upset.** If you must eat in a hurry, eat a very small meal. By eating slowly, the digestion catches up to the mouth. Many people who have lived over 100 years practice this fundamental rule: **Chew your food well** (20-40 times is optimum). Stop eating when you are full. If you practice the three meals and five snacks a day plan, you will feel fuller sooner. The Lazy Person's style of eating is based on enjoyment, not denial. No one likes a diet, because starvation is no fun. **Denial is not the way to health, nor is over-eating.**

Eat Natural Foods Whenever Possible

Other than whole grains, beans, nuts and seeds which are protected by an outer covering, wholesome, fresh, live food is very fragile and spoils if left on your kitchen counter overnight. **Eat foods which can spoil, decay and rot.** Most canned, frozen or otherwise processed foods contain additives for color, taste and preservation, making them potentially hazardous to our health. Read labels carefully and avoid chemical additives. Support your local health food stores and encourage the manager of your local grocery to develop a health food section within the store. Shopping at natural food stores will increase your knowledge of health and enable you to meet new friends. **The road to health has many nice people on it!**

Drink Before or After Meals

Drinking liquids with main meals dilutes your digestive juices and inhibits food digestion. Drink 30 minutes before or 30 mintues after a meal. Drinking near snacks will cause no digestive problems.

The Best Digestive Aid Is Exercise

Although daily exercise is essential to good digestion, do not eat immediately before or after intense physical or mental exertion. Read the Exercise Chapter for further guidelines.

Food Substitution

Nature abhors a vacuum. Whenever a vacuum is created, something will always fill it. Saying "no" to foods such as sugar, salt, fats and processed food will not accomplish the final goal of better health. "No" is not enough, "yes" is also required. Many people say to me, "I don't eat sugar, why am I having blood sugar problems?" Eliminating refined sugar only begins to solve the hypoglycemic problem. A person must also eat complex carbohydrates which provide the body with the necessary natural sugar. The Lazy Person's motto is: **"the**

easiest way to eliminate a bad habit is to develop a healthier one in its place." The replacement/substitution strategy will make the dietary transition easier.

Sweeteners

If grains and fruits are not enough to satisfy your "sweet tooth" at the beginning of your new diet, use Dr. Jensen's Apple Concentrate (syrup made from apples), barley malt syrup, or fruit juices such as pineapple, grape and apple for sweeteners. Barley malt and apple juice concentrate syrups can be added to bakery goods and plain yogurt.

Condiments

Black pepper, which is very irritating to the stomach lining, should be replaced with cayenne. Kelp, Vegit and Dr. Jensen's **Vegetable Broth** replace salt without eliminating the "salty" taste. Additionally, use Dr. Jensen's **Quick Sip** to replace tamari and soy sauce which are very high in salt content. Don't forget to experiment with herbs and spices when cooking (see list of herbs and spices in Chapter 1).

Most health food and grocery stores carry fresh herbs and information books to guide you in their use.

Salad Dressing

Natural salad dressings contain some honey and a little sea salt and are acceptable alternatives to commercial dressings. Olive oil and lemon are a wonderful addition to any salad. Create your own salad dressings in a blender using foods such as yogurt, avocado, lemon, herbs, apple cider vinegar and a salt substitute. When dining out, ask for vinegar and oil dressing which contains no salt or sugar.

Use only Unsalted Butter

Margarine is a processed food which is partially hydrogenated. In the processing of polyunsaturated oils, hydrogen is forced back into the molecular structure of fatty acids which makes the oil "solid" at room temperature. Oils in their natural state are liquid at room temperature. Our bodies have great difficulty breaking down hydrogenated oil which can cause arterial problems. Unsalted butter can be found in health food stores or in the "freezer section" of most supermarkets. It may safely be used in moderation (1 or 2 pats a day).

Nut Butters

Nut butters such as almond or sesame (tahini) are excellent substitutes for peanut butter on unsalted rye crisps or rice cakes. Raw, unsalted nut butter is best.

Coffee Substitutes

Cafix, Pero, Postum and other cereal coffees replace coffee, while herb teas replace commercial black teas which contain tannic acid and caffeine.

Alcoholic Beverages

If you must drink, dry white wine contains the least amount of sugar. Natural, lite beers are best. Fresh fruit and vegetable juices are a great substitute for alcoholic beverages. These juices give you a natural high with no hangover.

Lunch Meats

Avocado or guacamole, fish, natural chicken or turkey and nut butters are fine substitutes for highly processed luncheon meats.

Soups

Create your own homemade soup in a crock pot. Crock pots use low heat and don't require constant attention. Putting a cup or more of grains like brown rice, barley or millet into any soup makes a "hardier," thicker, delicious and more filling meal. Use rice flour or oat flour rather than wheat to thicken soups. Natural food cookbooks contain numerous recipes (see list in back of this book).

Bread

Eat 100% whole grains (millet, brown rice, buckwheat, barley, oats, etc.) to replace bread. Many people crave starch because it converts to sugar or glucose when digested. Whole grains satisfy starch cravings and provide slowly digesting sugar as well. If you must eat bread, 100% sourdough rye bread, unsalted rye crisps, rice cakes and corn tortillas may be substituted. Use rice flour, oat flour, soy flour or buckwheat flour as substitutes when bread recipes call for wheat flour.

Canned Foods

Fresh vegetables and fruits are preferable to frozen. In turn, frozen foods are preferable to canned foods. You waste your hard-earned money on canned foods. Canned food is dead food. How much life would you have left after spending time in a sealed can?

Herbs for Common Ailments

Common drugs such as aspirin, antacids, laxatives, cold remedies and cough syrups should be replaced with natural herbs in capsules, extracts, essences and tinctures. These herbs can be found at local health food stores. **Substitute herbs for drugs whenever possible.** Your local health food store carries herbal books which will provide advice regarding proper usage for common ailments. **Caution:** Herbal combinations are medicine and should be taken for specific problems and for specific lengths of time. You wouldn't continually take an aspirin to prevent a possible headache just as you shouldn't take herbal formulas, designed for special ailments, all the time.

Water

Growing evidence reveals that chemicals added to purify public water systems are dangerous and even cancer producing. Since water is essential to good health, consider drinking bottled water (see Chapter Six).

Spring water, low in sodium content, is the preferred bottled water. This water is sold in supermarkets and health food stores and distributed by private water companies. I recommend drinking distilled water for a cleansing period of three to six months only. If you wish to continue drinking distilled water after this initial cleansing period, add two tablespoons of sea water (Catelina Sea Water is best) per gallon for remineralization. Your local health food store should carry Catalina Sea Water or know where it may be purchased. An economical way to drink distilled water is to make your own! Many companies manufacture **home-distillers.**

I DO HAVE TIME

Many people insist they don't have time to be healthy. The following research puts this excuse to rest.

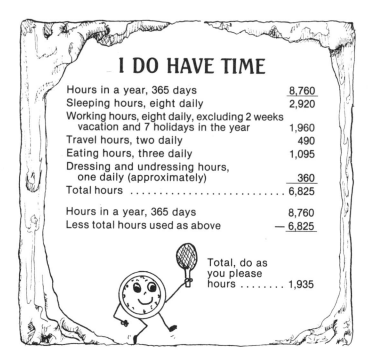

I DO HAVE TIME

Hours in a year, 365 days	8,760
Sleeping hours, eight daily	2,920
Working hours, eight daily, excluding 2 weeks vacation and 7 holidays in the year	1,960
Travel hours, two daily	490
Eating hours, three daily	1,095
Dressing and undressing hours, one daily (approximately)	360
Total hours	6,825
Hours in a year, 365 days	8,760
Less total hours used as above	— 6,825
Total, do as you please hours	1,935

All we need do is put our health first and utilize the "do as you please hours" for healthy purposes. Time is essential for eating, exercising regularly and healing properly. Fatigue, nervous exhaustion, sleeplessness and other symptoms you may be experiencing were not developed overnight. **Neither Rome nor a healthy lifestyle can be built in a day.** Patience is essential for healing.

Although we think we are saving time by eating fast foods, we are instead subtracting years off our lives. **How would you like to work all your life and not get paid?** Similarly, your body works very hard to digest the food you eat, only to discover that your diet is high in calories and low in supporting levels of vitamins, minerals and other essential nutrients. How long can your body work for no pay? **Remember, if you don't make time to be healthy, you are making time to be sick.**

BINGING — I CAN

"What many of us need most is a vigorous kick in the seat of our can'ts!"

When beginning a new diet, we have great expectations and inspiration. But there comes that day when we inevitably "go off" our diet and junk out. In a moment of weakness we will eat some junk foods we have been dreaming about for weeks. Our self-esteem slips during such binges and we beat ourselves up by saying, "Oh well, I blew it, it's all over; I'm a bad person. I just can't do anything right."

My suggestion to you is to include binging in your eating program. If your diet includes a chance to kick up your heels and eat things you don't normally eat, it will be easier to "stay on your diet." Generally diets are considered as a form of punishment because we stop eating the foods we enjoy. Actually, the word diet is derived from the Greek word, diaita, meaning "a manner of living" or way of life. The Lazy Person is not interested in changing his diet, but rather changing his lifestyle, to improve his health. Life is not something you can go on and off of. **Developing a healthy lifestyle requires consistency, not perfection.** Take a look at society's idea of success. It is much less than perfect. For instance, a successful batter has a batting average of .300. According to this average, the batter fails two out of every three times he comes to the plate. Another sports example involves football. A quarterback considered successful completes at least 50% of his passes. Although one out of every two passes are not complete, the quarterback is looked upon as very successful. If you improve your lifestyle by 50%, your performance is probably 100% better than before.

I want you to begin thinking, "I am succeeding" and keep that thought even when you fail. Thomas Edison, failed in 1000 consecutive experiments before he finally invented the light bulb. When asked, "How could you continue after so many failures?" he replied, "I don't consider those failures, I think of them as 1000 ways how not to make a light bulb." This is a successful attitude. Every experiment ending in failure provided Edison with another piece of the puzzle, ultimately leading to a successful invention. While developing your healthy lifestyle, begin to think, "I make all my failures and mistakes part of my ultimate success." These failures are part of the process leading us to ultimate victory.

In the 1982 New York marathon, one inspiring story was told about a woman who ran the race on crutches. It took her more than eleven hours to complete the race. She fell eleven times and **completed** the race in the dark of the night after everyone else had gone home. The importance of this story is that although she fell eleven times, she got up eleven times, finishing the marathon.

The Lazy Person includes food binges as part of his/her nutritonal lifestyle. Dr. Paavo Airola discovered that all the healthy cultures he studied, occasionally binged! He found that these cultures celebrated a festival or a religious holiday every thirty days during which time they ate and drank in excess. After the day of partying was over, the people returned to their wholesome diets.

THE LAZY PERSON'S GUIDE TO BETTER NUTRITION **includes one day a month when we can eat all the candy bars, pies, cakes, pizzas or any other foods we wish, and we eat them without any guilt.** A binge day once or twice a month will not undermine our health and may even prove to be beneficial.

ACID AND ALKALINE — KEEPING BALANCE IN YOUR BODY

By knowing your urine pH, you can understand what is happening in your digestive tract. The "p" stands for potential and the "H" stands for hydrogen. The pH measures the potential of a solution to attract hydrogen ions. The pH range starts at "0" and continues to "14". A ph below 7 is considered acid, the lower the number becomes the more acid the solution. A pH above 7 is said to be alkaline and the alkalinity increases as the number increases. The number 7 pH is considered neutral by the scientists.

The urine pH reveals many health related factors. A pH of 5.2 is a very acid condition and forces food to pass through the digestive stomach and intestines rapidly in order to avoid burning the walls. When food rapidly passes through the digestive system, sufficient time is not allowed for the body to absorb vitamins and minerals. **Minerals are not utilized when the body has an over-acid condition.** Zinc, manganese and chromium will not absorb properly, causing profound effects on insulin production, hormonal balance and blood glucose metabolism. Furthermore, oil-soluble vitamins A, D, E and K as well as water soluble vitamins C and B-complex are not assimilated in this environment. Each vitamin and mineral requires a specific pH, beyond which they are not properly assimilated. Some nutritionists have said, "You are what you eat." The actual statement should be **"You are what you assimilate."** When your pH is not in balance, organs and glands experience vitamin and mineral starvation.

Deficiency proceeds disease and **it is much easier to correct a deficiency than a disease.**

Most Americans' urine pH is 5.3 to 5.6 which is too acid for proper digestion and assimilation. People with over-acid pH readings frequently experience such symptoms as increased heart rate, dry skin, infrequent urination, diminished perspiration, hemorrhoids and hardening of the arteries.

One way to prevent disease and improve nutrient absorption is to balance the pH of the body, Find out what your urine pH is by following this simple procedure. Purchase nitrazine paper (range 04.5 pH to 7.5 pH) at a pharmacy. Eat your normal dinner and fast until morning (approximately 12 hours).

29

No juices, food, supplements or drugs should be ingested during the fasting period. Only water is permitted during the twelve-hour fast. Do not use the first urination of the morning as a sample since overnight detoxification makes the urine very acidic. Use the second or third urination of the morning and place the specimen in a paper cup. Dip approximately an inch of the nitrazine strip into the urine specimen and match the color with the color coding chart in the nitrazine kit. **The urine pH should read 6.3 to 6.5 after a twelve-hour overnight fast.** Repeat this procedure for three or four days to arrive at an average pH reading. If your pH is **below** 6.3, as is the case of most Americans, then your food is only partially digested, and therefore, only partially absorbed. If your pH is above 6.5 your urine is over-alkaline. The more alkaline your urine pH, the weaker the digestive juices become. Digestive enzymes are not strong enough to break down the food for assimilation. An alkaline system is a a sluggish and slow one. People with a high pH often experience stiff joints, muscle cramps, lowered resistance to viruses, bacteria, fungus (micro-organisms thrive in an alkaline environment), lung problems and constipation.

Healthy cultures eat a predominantly alkaline diet; 75% alkaline and only 25% acid. In America, the diet is just the reverse because of the high consumption of acid foods such as meat, dairy products and refined carbohydrates. The taste of a food has absolutely nothing to do with whether it is acid or alkaline; the ash which the food becomes within the body is the determining factor.

An alkaline-rich diet will correct an over-acid or over-alkaline system. If you have an acid condition in your digestive tract and you change your diet to predominantly alkaline foods, you may experience a lot of gas. This gas may continue for several days or weeks. When baking soda is placed on sulfuric acid it creates a fizzing chemical reaction. The same holds true when an alkaline diet is put into a body where an acid condition exists. Much bubbling, grumbling and flatulence is experienced. As the diet continues, less and less discomfort will be experienced.

The following is a list of acid and alkaline foods. By eating more alkaline foods and eating less meat, dairy and refined sugars, a person can improve the pH of the digestive tract.

ACID FOODS

Binging Foods Only

Sugars (processed)
Veal
Organ meats
Liver
Chicken
Turkey
Most muscle meats
Peanuts
Most nuts (except almonds)
White rice
Oysters
Shrimp
Crab
Lobster
Sardines
Rabbit
Beef
Pork
Bacon
Ham
Duck
Goose
Macaroni
White Bread
Black tea
Coffee
Crackers
Honey
Natural cheese

Acceptable

(25% of daily calories)
Poultry
Fish (fins & scales)
Eggs (not fried)
Natural grains (except
    millet and buckwheat)
Beans
Lentils and split peas
Rolled oats
Cranberries
Whole grain breads
    (in moderation)

ALKALINE FOODS (75% of daily calories)

Apples
Bananas
Peaches
Sweet plums
Grapes
Watermelon and seeds
Most fruit juices
Fig juice
Coconut
Pomegranate
Olives, green and ripe
Sweet chives
Raisins
Currents
Figs
Most herbal teas
Squash
Nectarines
Oranges
Grapefruit
Lemons
Almonds (especially
   almond milk)
Beets and beet greens
Dates
Apricots
Millet

Celery
Carrots
Cantaloupe
Parsley
Watercress
Pineapple
Tomatoes
Cabbage
Sweet potatoes
Potatoes, especially red
Lettuce (romaine, bibb, leaf)
Swiss chard
Rutabaga
Mushrooms
Parsnips
Radishes
Peas
Pears
Artichoke
Onions
String beans
Kale
Cauliflower
Asparagus
Endive
Buckwheat
Sprouting Seeds

*Overcooked vegetables become acid forming
 If fruits are eaten green they are acid forming

If blood sugar is low omit:
1. Dried fruit
2. Honey
3. Molasses
4. Grapes
5. Oranges

NEUTRAL FOODS
Yogurt (plain and unsweetened)

When the proper ratio of acid and alkaline foods is established (three parts alkaline and one part acid), strong resistance and immunity to disease will result. After a month on the improved alkaline-acid balanced diet, repeat the procedure for checking your pH. If there is no improvement, you have been acid for many years. Be patient. Since it took years to develop an over-acid condition, give yourself a few months to correct the pH.

HEALING CRISIS

Beginning a new exercise program after months of non-activity would probably cause stiffness, tiredness and aching throughout the body. These symptoms would be part of the process necessary in order to "get back in shape." Similarly, **in the initial three months of a new diet such symptoms as stiffness, skin rashes, aching muscles, weakness, nausea, tiredness, diarrhea and cold symptoms may be experienced.** These conditions are part of the natural cleansing process as stored toxins, drugs, waste products and other poisons are pulled out of the tissues and circulatory system. This cleansing process is natural and healthy and reflects your body's ability to "get back in nutritional condition" again. **Do not panic, the symptoms pass quickly (one day to a week usually).**

A Healing Crisis, as Dr. Jensen calls this phenomenon, happens when the body has built up enough vitality to stand the shock of the detoxification.

Sometimes the body eliminates the waste a little at a time, making a crisis unnecessary, but this is the exception, not the rule. **Rest and relaxation will enable your body to handle a healing crisis in the shortest possible time.**

CHAPTER 3

CARBOHYDRATES:
THE ENERGY YOUR BODY RUNS ON

"IF YOU DON'T KNOW WHERE YOU'RE GOING, ANY ROAD WILL TAKE YOU THERE." old saying

Carbohydrates have received "bad press" in newspapers, magazines and books in recent years. People have been led to believe that carbohydrates are fattening and should be avoided. However, only **refined carbohydrates are fattening** because they are high in calories and low in vitamins and minerals. **Foods increase in empty calories as they are processed.** For instance, potatoes are an excellent carbohydrate, rich in protein, energy and less than 1% fat. Potato chips, on the other hand, are processed until they become 40% fat! Potato chips should be renamed—Fat Chips.

POTATOES: THE GOOD, BAD & UGLY
per 100 grams (3½ oz.)

	CALORIES	FAT grams
BAKED 1 Potato	93	.1
FRENCH FRIES frozen, oven heated	220	8.4
CHIPS 10 each	568	39.8

Source: U.S. Department of Agriculture Handbook #8.

Carbohydrates are the preferred and finest source of energy for the human body. As a child, I was taught that protein was the best source of energy for my body. I accepted the following energy equation:

$$Energy = Protein$$
$$Protein = Meat \qquad \textbf{wrong}$$
$$Energy = Meat$$

Actually, the perfect source of fuel for most body functions including the brain, nerves and muscles is carbohydrates. Your energy is derived from **glucose,** or sugar, which **provides immediate energy.** Carbohydrates break down easily into glucose. The correct energy equation is:

$$Energy = Glucose$$
$$Glucose = Carbohydrates \qquad \textbf{right}$$
$$Energy = Carbohydrates$$

The human brain depends primarily on carbohydrates for its energy. Therefore, your attitude toward life is affected significantly by the brain's glucose supply.

The bottom line need for all body cells is energy. Carbohydrates are your body's first choice for energy every time. The absence of adequate carbohydrates in the diet causes the body to convert protein or fat into energy. Fats are stored in the fat cells of the body for future energy requirements while **carbohydrates are designed for immediate energy requirements.** If fat is converted into glucose instead of stored, the result is inferior energy which cannot be used efficiently by the brain or central nervous system. **In the absence of adequate carbohydrates, the body will devalue protein, and convert it into glucose.**

PROTEIN'S USES IN THE BODY

1. Maintenance and repair of cells
2. Hormone production
3. Enzymes for use in digestion
4. Anti-bodies to fight infection

These vital protein functions **are sacrificed** in order to manufacture glucose when insufficient carbohydrates are eaten. The conversion of protein into glucose is a costly one. Here is what happens. The liver is forced to remove the amine group (nitrogen group) from the protein and send it to the kidneys in the form of urea. The kidneys must then work harder to remove the excess urea by excreting it out of the body via the urine. **Using protein instead of carbohydrates for energy is the same as using dollar bills to start a fire instead of newspaper.** High protein, low carbohydrate weight loss diets advocated by so-called nutritionists are damaging to both the liver and kidneys and threaten to upset the hormonal balance, the immune system and the rebuilding of cells in an otherwise normal person. One may experience weight loss with a high protein, low carbohydrate diet because the body is **starving** without the needed carbohydrates. **A low carbohydrate intake can cause symptoms of protein deficiency.** Therefore, if the body is forced to use protein instead of the preferred carbohydrate, bodily functions for which protein are crucial will not be adequately performed.

Carbohydrates in the form of starch have been the ideal source of human energy for centuries. A human's large brain requires a high glucose diet (found in starch) which provides warmth and fuel. The discovery and cultivation of grains provided this slow-acting glucose, allowing man to concentrate his brain power upon things other than hunting and gathering food. **Humans have lived primarily on complex carbohydrates for thousands of years.**

> Rice - 12,000 years
> Beans, squash - 9,000 years
> Wheat, barley - 7,000 years
> Table sugar - 100 years

Besides containing glucose for energy, grains have vitamins needed to operate the brain, the nervous system, the immune glands (pituitary, thyroid, adrenals) and the neuromuscular system.

MAKE-UP OF A KERNEL OF GRAIN
Oats, brown rice, millet, barley, buckwheat, rye, cornmeal.

ENDOSPERM (83%)

GERM (2½%)

BRAN (14%)

HULL

TOTAL NUTRIENTS IN A KERNEL OF GRAIN

GERM	BRAN	ENDOSPERM
Thiamine (B¹)	Pyridoxine (B⁶)	Starch
Riboflavin (B²)	Panthothenic Acid	Traces of
Pyridoxine (B⁶)	(B⁵)	Vitamins &
Protein	Riboflavin (B²)	Minerals
Pantothenic Acid	Thiamine (B¹)	
(B⁵)	Protein	
Niacin (B³)		
Vitamin E		

MINERALS

Calcium	Sulphur	Barium
Iron	Iodine	Silver
Phosophorus	Fluorine	Inositol
Magnesium	Chlorine	Folic Acid
Potassium	Sodium	Choline
Manganese	Silicon	And other trace
Copper	Boron	materials

Source: Nutrition Almanac

If we examine the structure of any grain, seed or nut, four distinctive parts are found: the husk, the bran, the germ and the endosperm. **The husk** is a protective covering with little nutritional value. **The bran** is primarily insoluble fiber called cellulose, containing small amounts of B-vitamins, minerals (especially iron) and protein. **The endosperm,** constituting the largest part of the grain, is mostly starch, incomplete protein and trace amounts of nutrients. **The germ** is the center or heart of a grain, seed, or nut, and is **especially** rich in B-vitamins, Vitamin E, protein, unsaturated fat, minerals and carbohydrates. Even though the carbohydrate known as starch is a rich source of glucose (energy), **the germ and bran portion contains the B-vitamins and minerals necessary for the digestion of the starch in the endosperm.** The bran and the germ are generally removed during the milling process to eliminate possible rancidity and increase the shelf life of the grain. Thus a complex carbohydrate becomes a refined carbohydrate. **Most of the grains we eat in the U.S. contain only the endosperm or starchy element** which is constipating and practically indigestible without the bran and germ. These refined grains are fattening. Carbohydrates are not all the same, just as there are different forms of transportation. Although a pogo stick and a bicycle are both forms of transportation, one is more efficient than the other. A potato and a potato chip are both carbohydrates, but one contains empty calories and little nutritional value while the other is well used by the body. **Calories don't count, but the type of calorie does.**

Grains, such as oats, millet, barley, rice, wheat and corn, supply over 50% of human energy for every man, woman and child on the earth (see Chapter 1).

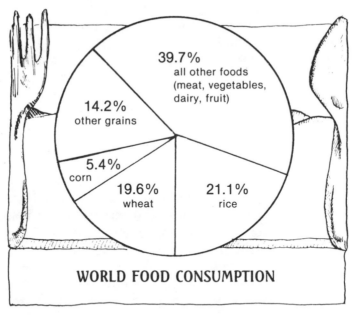

WORLD FOOD CONSUMPTION

39.7%
all other foods
(meat, vegetables,
dairy, fruit)

14.2%
other grains

5.4%
corn

19.6%
wheat

21.1%
rice

Source: Nutrition Concepts & Controversies

Complex carbohydrates, especially grains, are so essential to human health that the Select Committee on Nutrition and Human Needs, United States Senate, investigated the nutritional habits of people all over the world, and made a recommendation regarding carbohydrates. In the report entitled **Dietary Goals for the United States,** the Committee suggested to "increase carbohydrate consumption to account for 55% to 60% of the energy (caloric) intake in the American diet." The government's recommendation to increase our carbohydrate consumption is an official acknowledgement of its importance, and yet, the use of grains in the U.S. has been declining.

COMPARISON OF GRAIN CONSUMPTION for U.S. 1910 – 1976		
GRAIN	1910 Per Capita	1976 Per Capita
RYE	3.6 lbs down	.8 lbs
BARLEY	3.5 lbs down	1.2 lbs
BUCKWHEAT	2.1 lbs down	.05 lbs
CORNMEAL	51.1 lbs down	7.7 lbs
OATMEAL	3-4 lbs same	3-4 lbs
RICE	7.2 lbs same	7.2 lbs

Source: *Changing American Diet* by the Center for Science in the Public Interest.

FIBER IN GRAINS

Recently, many authorities have advocated that by increasing dietary fiber, especially bran, a person can improve elimination. Dietary fiber, including cellulose, and hemicelluloses, is an indigestible bulk which massages the walls of the colon. The "broom" effect of fiber increases stool size and reduces transit time. Colon cancer is diagnosed in over 90,000 people a year in the U.S. and kills 60,000. Next to lung cancer, colon cancer is the deadliest. A diet high in fat (the U.S. diet contains 40-50% fat) forces the liver and gallbladder to produce excess bile acids. Recent studies conclude that a high concentration of bile acids caused by high fat intake irritate the colon wall, leaving it more vulnerable to cancer-causing agents. Both Finnish and American cultures consume a high fat diet, yet the Finns have much lower rates of colon cancer. The difference seems to be the higher fiber diets among Finns which dilutes the deadly bile acids. Clinical studies on colon cancer conclude: 1) reducing the amount of fat in the diet also reduces the amount of bile acids in the stool, and 2) increasing the amount of dietary fiber or roughage in the diet increases the volume of the stool, diluting concentration of bile acids. Colon cancer is preventable.

In the healthy cultures high complex carbohydrate/low fat diets were the rule. All cultures studied were free of colon cancer. Whole grains, such as oats, barley, rice, corn, rye, buckwheat and millet, are the best sources of bran (dietary fiber) and are protective foods against constipation, diverticulosis, irritable bowel syndrome and colon cancer. Beans and starchy vegetables like carrots and squash are also protective foods.

The average number of stools (bowel movements) **in healthy cultures is two-three a day;** in the United States one or less is common. If you are eating two or three meals a day and are experiencing only one bowel movement a day, you are constipated! Eating whole grains, rich in needed fiber, once or twice a day will increase stool volume and transit time. Food fiber should be increased gradually so as not to provoke intolerances. A daily intake of 25 grams of fiber is recommended and assured when a person follows the Optimum Diet for Optimum Health.

In general, 1. a serving of whole, cooked vegetables is 2 grams of fiber (eat 4 servings a day) 2. a serving of 1/2 cup cooked grains is 2 grams of fiber (eat 1-2 servings a day) 3. 1 slice whole grain bread, or 2 rye crackers is 2 grams of fiber (as needed) 4. a medium whole fruit is 2 grams of fiber (eat two a day). Since insoluble fiber found in grains is a prime cancer fighter, The Lazy Person's Guide recommends **"You Rough It."***

*Although many nutrition experts lump all the fiber foods together — **whole grains and beans are the superior and preferred fiber to eat, followed by vegetables.**

CARBOHYDRATES AND BLOOD SUGAR

For years, diabetics have been placed on a restricted carbohydrate diet and told to avoid sugar and starch. Many recent studies demonstrate that blood glucose control improves and insulin requirements decrease with a high-carbohydrate, high fiber, low fat diet. Whole grains, beans and vegetables are slow-digesting sugars or polysaccharides, releasing energy (glucose) much the same as a time-released vitamin supplement. **Digestion of polysaccharides such as grains takes four to six hours. Sugars enter the bloodstream on a continuous basis and stabilize blood sugar for hours.** Since large amounts of insulin are not required as is the case with concentrated and refined sugar, **complex carbohydrates actually lower insulin demands.**

After a person eats a breakfast of oatmeal, a steady, stable energy level will be felt for several hours due to the time-released sugar quality of the oats. (Other grains act this way, too.)

Complex carbohydrates are the slow-digesting glucose your body needs to maintain consistent energy and win the Energy Game. The vitamin, mineral and high fiber content of whole grains, beans, seeds, and nuts makes their consistent use a must for the Lazy Person who eats to live. A diet high in complex carbohydrates helps you break the refined sugar habit by giving your brain and body the natural sugar it needs to function optimally. Cakes, pies, cookies and candy will become less and less a part of your life as more and more grains and vegetables are eaten.

CHAPTER 4

PROTEIN:
HOW MUCH IS ENOUGH?

"AS LONG AS YOU LIVE, KEEP LEARNING HOW TO LIVE."
Greek saying

A baby triples its weight in the first year of life, growing from seven to 21 pounds! Since protein is necessary for growth one would think a baby's incredible increase in size means there is a substantial percentage of protein in mother's milk. **Actually, nature provides only 3-6% protein in human milk!** During a period of your life when protein is in great demand you're on a diet that provides 3-6%. We need far less protein than we think. **According to the Recommended Daily Allowance for protein, the older we become the less protein we require. By the time we reach 19 years old, our protein requirement is only .8 grams per 2.2 pounds of ideal body weight and remains consistent for the rest of our lives.** If you feel you are at your ideal body weight (or refer to height, weight, sex, age chart), divide that weight by 2.2 pounds. For instance, if I weighed 110 lbs., I would divide 110 by 2.2 which works out to 50. If I multiply .8 grams times 50, I have an answer of 40 grams. A 110–pound person needs 40 grams of protein per day unless pregnant or lactating. If you are pregnant add 30 grams of protein; if you are lactating add 20 grams of protein.

In healthy cultures of the world, the average protein intake is 30-60 grams per adult per day. The RDA for the average adult in the United States is 45 grams, a figure very consistent with the quantity of protein eaten in healthy cultures. **Most Americans eat two to three times the quantity of protein required by the RDA (45 grams) to maintain protein balance.** For instance, a Standard American Diet (S.A.D.) for breakfast is 2 eggs, a 3-ounce slice of ham or bacon, a glass

45

of milk and 2 slices of toast, which contribute 47 grams of protein. An average breakfast alone would provide adequate protein for an entire day.

The S.A.D. for lunch would be a quarter pound of hamburger with a slice of cheese, totaling 40 grams of protein. This amount almost qualifies as enough for the entire day.

Since meat is a favorite protein of Americans, such a dish for dinner is a likely choice. Steak and potatoes (8 oz. steak and one medium potato) provide 58 grams of protein. **Computing the protein content of "three-squares" a day in the above mentioned menu provides 145 grams of protein.** This hypothetical, but not unrealistic, menu constitutes three times as much protein as the RDA requirement!

There are very definite risks associated with the overconsumption of protein:

1. **Diets high in protein increase the body's loss of calcium** (ratio of calcium to phosphorous in meat is 1:20 rather than the ideal of 2:1). Excess phosphorous depletes calcium.

2. **The higher a person's intake of meat and dairy, the more fruits, vegetables and grains will be crowded out of the diet, causing important nutrient deficiencies.**

3. **Because the human body has no adequate system for eliminating large quantities of excess protein, the liver and kidneys overwork to accommodate the overload (protein overload effect).**

4. **Excess protein accumulates on the walls of the tiny capillaries leading to cells, reducing the capillaries' ability to give adequate nutrients to the individual cells (cell starvation).**

5. **Excess protein is accompanied by large amounts of fat associated with a high risk of atherosclerosis or hardening of the arteries.**

The fifth point establishes the relationship between protein foods such as meat and high fat content. Although most people believe meat is a protein food, further study reveals a surprising fact. **A quarter-pound hamburger, mentioned as being the average lunch of many Americans, contains 28 grams of protein and 23 grams of fat.** Because fat offers twice as many calories per gram as protein, a hamburger contains 112 calories of protein and 207 calories of fat! Consequently, **con-**

sumers of high meat diets tend to be overweight.

Poultry and fish provide a high protein source with a lower fat content than meat. The Lazy Person's Guide strongly recommends a drastic reduction (once a month is enough) of all meat (beef, pork, veal, luncheon meats, ham and bacon) and the substitution of fresh poultry and fish. Both fish and poultry have high concentrations of protein. For example, four ounces of cooked salmon contains 27 grams of protein, and four ounces of roasted chicken contains 31 grams of protein: **The Lazy Person's Guide recommends eating fish and poultry less frequently and in smaller portions.** When fish is eaten three days a week and poultry once a week, additional grains, vegetables and fruits can be consumed to provide more complex carbohydrates, fiber, vitamins and minerals for energy.

Substituting whole grains for fish and poultry will also supply complete protein to your diet. Grains, beans and legumes are often called the "Poor Man's Meat." Most Americans believe the only "complete" proteins are meat, fish, poultry, eggs and dairy products, assuming the vegetable kingdom contains only "incomplete" proteins. To the nutritionist, an "incomplete" protein is a food totally lacking in one or more of the essential amino acids. Few foods are in that category.

ESSENTIAL AMINO ACID CONTENT per 100 grams (3½ oz.)

in milligrams

	TRYPTO-PHAN	THREO-NINE	ISOLEU-CINE	LEU-CINE	LYSINE	METH-IONINE	PHENY-LALANINE	VALINE	HISTI-DINE	PROTEIN GRAMS
GRAINS										
BARLEY	160	433	545	889	433	184	661	643	239	8.2
CORN (field whl)	61	398	462	1,296	288	186	454	510	206	8.9
MILLET	248	456	635	1,746	383	270	506	682	240	9.9
RICE, brown	81	294	352	646	296	135	377	524	126	7.5
RYE, whl grain	137	448	515	813	494	191	571	631	276	12.1
LEGUMES										
PINTO BEANS	213	997	1,306	1,976	1,708	232	1,270	1,395	655	22.9
LENTILS	216	896	1,316	1,760	1,528	180	1,104	1,360	548	24.7
NUTS/SEEDS										
ALMONDS	176	610	873	1,454	582	259	1,146	1,124	514	18.6
PECANS	138	389	553	773	435	153	564	525	273	9.2
SUNFLOWER	343	911	1,276	1,736	868	443	1,220	1,354	586	24.0

Source: Amino Acid Content of Foods, Home Economics Research Report #4, U.S. Department of Agriculture, 1968.

48

Protein is found in both plants and animals. Protein consists of 21 amino acids connected in chains. The length and sequence of the amino acid chains distinguish one type of protein from another. Of the 21 amino acids, nine cannot be produced within the body (called essential amino acids) and must therefore be included in your diet. These nine amino acids are: tryptophane, histine, phenylalanine, leucine, isoleucine, valine, lysine, threonine and methionine. Eggs are considered the only food which has the "ideal" balance of essential amino acids needed by humans. The egg is the reference point or standard against which all other proteins are measured. Although vegetable proteins compared with egg protein are lower in quantity of essential amino acids, the real standard of protein is its quality. Quality refers to the amino acids' usability by the human body. If vegetable and animal proteins are considered in terms of quality, there is little difference between the two classes of proteins. Since most of the healthy cultures use little or no animal protein in their diets and have no amino acid deficiencies, perhaps the egg, "the ideal reference protein," contains amino acids in excess of human requirements. **Although an egg may be the Rolls-Royce of proteins, vegetable proteins provide more than adequate essential amino acids to maintain optimum health.**

Since most complex carbohydrates contain all the essential amino acids, **complimentary protein meals to approximate the ideal pattern of amino acids in an egg is unnecessary.**

The fundamental difference between proteins and the other two food groups, carbohydrates and fats, is nitrogen. A method for measuring the amount of nitrogen retained by the body was standardized by the Food and Agriculture Organization of the United States. **The higher the percentage of nitrogen retained by the body, the higher the quality of the protein.** The result of these measurements is called **Biological Value.** The most perfect protein by this standard is egg protein. A biological value of 70% or above makes the quality of protein acceptable.

Egg - 94% B.V.
Fish - 74-90% B.V.

Millet - 88% B.V.
Brown Rice - 86% B.V.

A person need not be concerned about lack of adequate protein if he begins to eat less meat, fish or poultry. Meat, dangerously high in fat, provides no fiber; whereas grains, legumes and beans contain significant amounts of fiber.

Although protein deficiencies are almost unheard of in the United States, protein excesses are commonplace. The harmful effects of excess protein are well-documented. **THE LAZY PERSON'S GUIDE TO BETTER NUTRITION, encourages readers to reduce total fat and protein intake by half.** This reduction is most easily accomplished by eliminating red meats (beef, pork, veal). **Eat poultry and fish a few times a week and add whole grains, legumes and beans generously to your diet.**

HIGH PROTEIN AND WEIGHT LOSS

The functions of protein include: hormone production, antibody manufacturing, cell growth and repair, and enzyme production. **Only protein** can perform all the functions described above, but will be used as such only if the protein-sparing calories supplied by carbohydrates adequately meet the body's energy needs. Sacrificing protein requirements in order to create energy may result in nutritional deficiencies such as hormonal imbalances, allergies, malabsorption, improper healing of wounds, hypoglycemia and diabetes.

The Lazy Person's Guide questions those so-called "experts" who advocate high protein (meat), liquid protein or powdered protein weight loss programs while reducing important carbohydrate intake. Such high protein/low carbohydrate diets are unhealthy and eventually result in **obesity.** High protein diets induce only temporary weight loss (95% of people who lose weight regain it). Research indicates that carbohydrates, not protein, increase Dietary-Induced Thermogenesis (DIT). **The rate at which your body burns calories is boosted by DIT,** a metabolic process beginning after meals and continuing around the clock. **Carbohydrates excelerate the DIT, thus calories consumed as carbohydrates lead to less fat storage than calories eaten as protein.**

Eating the **Optimum Diet For Optimum Health,** high in complex carbohydrates, low in protein will insure a safe, healthy and permanent weight loss. To the Lazy Person, "Where's the beef?", is of no concern since he is more likely to ask "Where's the beans?"

CHAPTER 5

FOOD SUPPLEMENTS: ADDING INSURANCE TO YOUR DIET

"WHERE THERE IS NO VISION, THE PEOPLE PERISH."
Proverbs 29:18

There are those in the nutrition field who insist that food supplements are unnecessary. Food supplements consist of vitamins, minerals, and herbs (in pill, powder or liquid form) which are added to a diet to enhance the nutrient content of food. Those opposed to vitamin and mineral supplementation argue that if a diet is "well balanced," a person will obtain all the vitamins and minerals needed to maintain good health. Ideally, we should be able to eat a healthy diet and absorb all the protein, carbohydrates, fats, vitamins and minerals which our bodies need for optimum health. However, there are many factors that make this ideal impossible.

The quality of food grown in the United States even 30 years ago was superior to the nutritional content of foods today. The age of **Chemical Farming** is here. Extensive use of synthetic fertilizers, fungicides, pesticides and herbicides produce foods of inferior and questionable quality. Furthermore, processing and refining of many foods in order to increase shelf life, removes valuable vitamins, minerals and enzymes from already depleted grains, vegetables and fruits.

Most people today live in close proximity to thousands of others. Whether we are spectators at sporting events, watching a movie at a local theater or shopping in a large mall, **we are exposed to many more viruses and germs than people of past generations.** Our immune systems must cope with this bombardment of viruses; and in order to protect us, the need for vitamins and minerals, such as B-complex, C, A, calcium, magnesium, zinc and potassium, are in greater demand today than at any other time in history.

Modern western man, living on a diet of refined foods and maintaining a lifestyle of high stress, has developed many vitamin and mineral deficiencies. Most of us are second or third generation processed and junk food users. These "plastic" foods not only are deficient in vital nutrients needed to support us, but deplete our bodies of vitamins and minerals already stored.

Reasons for taking supplements are:
1. The poor quality of foods grown in depleted soil.
2. Modern refining and processing of foods.
3. Urban crowding which increases exposure to viruses and infection.
4. Mental and emotional stresses of urban living.
5. Constant exposure to air pollutants, chemicals and other carcinogenic substances in the environment.
6. Inherited vitamin and mineral deficiencies.

MINERALS

Without a proper mineral balance, our bodies cannot absorb and hold vitamins. You can take all the vitamin supplements on the market, but without the minerals which are the building blocks of health, you will never feel really well. Before vitamins, before man, the ancient earth was composed of inorganic minerals. Pre-historic plant life utilized and transformed these inorganic minerals, which animals could not assimilate, into the organic forms they could. Today, we eat both the plants and the animals in order to obtain our precious organic minerals. As we study nature and life processes, we arrive at one inexorable conclusion: the smaller the element, the more powerful its consequences. Atoms, invisible to the human eye when split, can annihilate the world. Although minerals make up only a small percentage of our bodies (5%), they determine our health to a large degree. Minerals help our cells function optimally, harden our teeth and bones, assist in digestion and hormone production, and are catalysts in such biological reactions as muscle response, transmission of message along the nerves and utilization of nutrients in foods. Without minerals we would be unable to maintain fluid balance, maintain acid-alkaline balance, transport nutrients into, around and out of the cells, and produce antibodies for proper immunity.

Refined foods, mineral poor soils and over-cooking have contributed to the mineral poor diets of most Americans. Nutritionists realize that many degenerative diseases originate as a result of one or more mineral deficiencies.

CALCIUM

Calcium is probably the most common mineral deficiency in America today. **Over-consumption of refined sugar, coffee, fat, alcohol and red meats, as well as stress, are the major causes of calcium deficiencies.**

Approximately 99% of all the calcium in the body is found in the bones and teeth. The bones and teeth act as reservoirs where calcium can be deposited or withdrawn as needed.

Roles of Calcium
1. Important in nerve transmission.
2. Builds and maintains bones and teeth.
3. Required for muscle contraction.
4. Helps regulate the heart beat.
5. Aids in iron utilization.
6. A catalyst for many metabolic functions.
7. Assists in process of blood clotting.
8. Helps maintain acid-alkaline balance in blood.
9. Regulates nutrients in and out of cells.

Calcium needs to combine with magnesium, phosphorus, and/or vitamins A, C and D for proper utilization. Hormones, not food, regulate calcium's absorption. Approximately 30% of ingested calcium is absorbed; the rest is excreted in the stool. **A high fat diet inhibits the absorption of calcium.** Fat binds the calcium into a soapy material which is excreted in the feces.

Symptoms of Calcium Deficiency
Symptoms include rickets, osteomalacia (adult rickets), osteoporosis, arthritis, muscle cramps, nervous afflictions, numbness and tingling in hands and feet, "popping bones," joint pains, headaches, tooth decay, insomnia, heart palpatations and many more.

Calcium helps regulate nerve transmission, and consequently, nervousness, hyperactivity, impatience, headaches, restlessness and sleeplessness are important signs of calcium deficiency. **Calcium is known as "the lullaby mineral"** because of its relaxing, calming and soothing effect on the nervous system. Calcium also buffers and neutralizes acid in the body. Symptoms of burning in the stomach and excessive gas and belching due to an over-acidic condition can be caused by lack of calcium. Stiffness, swollen or aching joints, and bones that make cracking sounds are other signs of calcium deficiency. If you have a history of dental decay, calcium is missing.

For Best Calcium Absorption

Magnesium is necessary for the proper absorption of calcium. **Taking calcium exclusively depletes the magnesium needed for proper function of muscles, particularly the heart.** Many vitamin manufacturers combine calcium and magnesium in one tablet. Calcium-magnesium supplemnts are combined in a ratio of two parts calcium to one part magnesium. **However, calcium and magnesium compete for the same pathways of absorption in the body, and in large dosages, neutralize each other.**

For best assimilation of calcium and magnesium, take them separately. Calcium should be taken before bed on an empty stomach, while magnesium is best absorbed with food during the day. The proper ratio of calcium to magnesium (2 to 1) is maintained by taking 1,000 mg. of calcium at bedtime and 500 mg. of magnesium at breakfast or lunch.

Calcium loss is more rapid among females than males for various reasons. Menstration, pregnancy and estrogen depletion all contribute to greater demands for calcium among women. Women may take 1,500 mg. of calcium and 750 mg. of magnesium daily before menopause. After menopause the amount of the hormone estrogen decreases and calcium demand increases. Post-menopausal women need to take 1,000 mg. of calcium at bedtime and another 1,000 mg. of calcium in the morning. Magnesium for post-menopausal women should be 500 mg. at the breakfast meal and another 500 mg. at the lunch or dinner meal.

Supplementation

Dolomite is a rock and is not very usable by humans (potential lead toxicity)

Bone Meal - humans don't digest bones well (potential lead toxicity)

Oyster Shell - shells do not assimilate well in humans

Calcium Lactate - good source if not allergic to milk

Calcium Gluconate - good source

Calcium Orotate - over priced, but good source

Calcium Chelate - Caution - chelation **forces** the body to accept this form. Use only if **severely** deficient.

Note: When taking calcium, a magnesium deficiency may result unless magnesium is also taken. Remember the 2 to 1 ratio 1,000 mg. calcium - 500 mg. magnesium.

Food Sources of Calcium

Nuts and seeds - almonds, chia seeds, sesame seeds, brazil nuts, filberts

Whole grains - barley, beans, brown rice, buckwheat, millet, oats, rye, lentils, cornmeal (yellow)

Vegetables - brussel sprouts, broccoli, cauliflower, parsnips, onions, green vegetables, avocadoes, carrots

Fish

Egg Yolks

Dairy - Yogurt is best

Sea Vegetables - kelp, dulse, agar-agar

Americans consume large amounts of milk products (25% of entire U.S. diet), rich in calcium, yet widespread calcium deficiency in the population is found. Why? **Most of us do not digest milk products well because we lack the digestive enzyme lactase or we have an intolerance to the protein, casein, found in cow's milk** (read Chapter Nine for further explanation). An alternative calcium source to indigestable milk products is almonds.

COMPARISON: ALMOND vs. MILK (3½ oz.)

NUTRIENT	ALMOND Raw Unsalted	*COW'S MILK 3.5% fat	COW'S MILK 3.7% fat	*SKIM MILK
CALCIUM	234mg	118mg	117mg	121mg
PROTEIN	18.6mg	3.5mg	3.5mg	3.6mg
FIBER	2.6mg	0	0	0
PHOSPHORUS	504mg	93mg	92mg	95mg
IRON	4.7mg	trace	trace	trace
POTASSIUM	773mg	144mg	140mg	145mg
THIAMINE	.24mg	.03mg	.03mg	.04mg
RIBOFLAVIN	.92mg	.17mg	.17mg	.18mg

*Pasteurized and raw
Source: U.S. Department of Agriculture Handbook #8.

Almonds, raw and unsalted, contain more calcium than the same quantity of milk. **Why not eat more almonds to make up a calcium deficiency?** Although almonds do provide excellent dietary calcium to keep the body in calcium balance, one would have to eat twenty or thirty pounds of almonds a day for several months or years to make up a deficiency. This solution is impractical, if not dangerous and unhealthy. A calcium supplement is the best way to make up a deficiency.

POTASSIUM

Potassium constitutes .0225% of the total mineral content of the body and is found primarily in the intracellular fluid.

Potassium is **critical to maintain heart beat. Other important tasks of potassium are:**

Roles of Potassium

1. Muscle contraction
2. Maintains proper alkalinity of the body fluids
3. Carries off fluids in lymphatic gland congestion
4. Regulates water balance
5. Assists in conversion of glucose to glycogen (sugar stored in liver)
6. Stimulates kidneys to eliminate body wastes
7. With phosphorous sends oxygen to the brain
8. With calcium regulates neuromuscular activity.

Potassium deficiency affects the brain cells early, and a person may not be aware of the deficiency until damage has already been done.

Deficiencies of potassium are caused by excessive intake of sodium chloride (salt), lack of adequate fruits and vegetables in the diet, profuse sweating for many days without adequate replacement, prolonged diarrhea and consumption of refined sugar, which causes large amounts of potassium to be used up in glucose metabolism. If potassium deficiency continues, muscles will not receive the energy needed and paralysis could result.

Symptoms of Potassium Deficiency

General weakness, impairment of nerves, muscle damage, poor reflexes, sagging muscles, memory loss, dizziness, confusion, constipation, slow and irregular heartbeat, carbohydrate intolerance, swelling and water retention.

Supplementation

A potassium complex of 99 mg. is the common supplement in health food stores and supermarkets.

A potassium supplement may be necessary for three to six months (100-200 mg. daily) if a high salt and/or sugar intake has been maintained for several years. After several months on potassium, a diet high in grains, fruits and vegetables coupled with an elimination of salt should be adequate to maintain potassium levels.

Food Sources

Nuts and seeds - almonds, anise seeds, walnuts, sunflower seeds, sesame seeds, pecans
Grains and Beans - lentils, pinto beans, brown rice, lima beans
Vegetables - potatoes, Jerusalem artichokes, carrots, parsley, watercress, broccoli, tomatoes, leaf lettuce, celery, spinach
Fruits - bananas, dates, currants, grapes, oranges, peaches, apples, watermelon, apricots, blueberries
Fish - All scaled fish

Bananas are excellent sources of natural potassium, but we would have to eat one hundred bananas a day for several months to replace the potassium losses due to salt alone. **The over-consumption of natural foods is not the answer to mineral deficiencies.** A complexed potassium supplement of 200 mg. a day, taken with meals for several months will improve this very dangerous deficiency.

VITAMIN PROTECTION

A common misconception regarding vitamins is that they provide energy. **Vitamins contain no energy within themselves.** Vitamins are coenzymes. Coenzymes are small molecules that combine with inactive protein to make an active enzyme. **Thanks to vitamins, which make protein enzymes active, energy is released from foods.** The energy of foods comes primarily from carbohydrates which break down into glucose for immediate use (see Chapter Three).

VITAMIN A

Vitamin A is a fat soluble nutrient naturally occurring in two forms. Pro-vitamin A, or carotene, is converted into Vitamin A by the body and found in the yellow, orange and green pigments of plants. The second form of Vitamin A is concentrated in animal tissues where the animal has metabolized the carotene contained in plant foods.

Roles of Vitamin A

Vitamin A aids in the growth and repair of body tissues, maintains smooth, soft skin and is essential in the formation of visual purple, a substance in the eye necessary for proper night vision.

Vitamin A has been called the anti-infection vitamin because it helps protect the mucous membranes of the nose, mouth, throat, lungs, stomach, intestines, urinary tract, bladder and vagina from infection. Without Vitamin A, cells are unable to secrete enough mucous to protect them from invading bacteria and infection. This protection also aids the mucous membranes in combating the effects of various air pollutants.

Symptoms of Vitamin A Deficiency

Signs of deficiency include lost of taste, night blindnes, infections, dry and aged skin, acne, sties in eyes and frequent fatigue.

Supplementation

Since people living in cities with high air-pollution are more susceptible to infections and colds than those in cleaner air environments, Vitamin A becomes a **must vitamin.** Since Vitamin A is fat soluble, however, it can be stored in the tissues of the body, making it potentially toxic. Taking fish-oil Vitamin A supplementation forces the body to either utilize the vitamin or store the excess.

To lessen the potential danger of Vitamin A toxicity, take the carotene form instead of fish oil. The conversion of carotene into Vitamin A is only 50% at best. Unabsorbed carotene is excreted in the urine. Since the body has a choice with carotene and no choice with fish oil, the preferred and safest supplementation of Vitamin A is carotene. Supplementing 10,000 I.U. to 30,000 of beta-carotene per day will permit your body to absorb up to 50% and excrete the rest.

Food Sources of Vitamin A

Fish, dairy, carrots, apricots, green leafy vegetables and broccoli.

B-COMPLEX

The B-complex family is essential for the release of energy from foods, to support the immune system and maintain the functions of the brain and nervous system.

Roles of B-Complex

1. Breaks down carbohydrates into glucose
2. Essential to brain function
3. Essential to healthy nervous system
4. Improves assimilation of foods
5. Helps convert glycogen of liver into energy
6. Supports the adrenal glands and thyroid functions

Complex carbohydrates, such as grains, contain significant amounts of B-complex which help release the glucose from the carbohydrate. The refining process, however, removes the B-vitamins from carbohydrates like white sugar and flour, forcing your body to take B-vitamins from the nervous system in order to have coenzymes. **The average American is severely deficient in the important B-vitamins, indispensable to the brain and the nervous system.**

Symptoms of B-Complex Deficiency

Nausea, exhaustion, tenderness and weakness in muscles, skin disorders, cracks in corners of mouth, swollen tongue, loss of memory, poor digestion, diarrhea, depression, oily skin, pernicious anemia, brain damage and paralysis.

Besides B-vitamin deficiencies caused by refined foods, a wide variety of drugs and medications also enhance deficiencies. Aspirin, oral contraceptives, alcohol, narcotics and anticonvulsants are only a few of the numerous drugs that contribute to B-vitamin depletion. The stress of modern living takes a great toll on the nerves, glands and hormones, all requiring B-family supplementation. Stress (see Chapter Ten), increases the need for B-vitamins.

Next to B-complex injections, sublingual (under the tongue) B-complex is the best form for immediate absorption into the bloodstream.

Food Sources of B-Complex
Whole grains, rice polishings (2 T in food), Fish

VITAMIN C
Vitamin C, like B-vitamins, is an example of a nutrient needed to fight the stresses of daily living and protect the body against disease. **Vitamin C is not stored or manufactured by the human body.**

Roles of Vitamin C
Vitamin C is necessary for the production and maintenance of collagen, a protein substance forming the base for all connective tissue. The formation of cellulite, according to some authorities, is a Vitamin C deficiency. Collagen heals wounds, mends fractures and prevents bruises. **Vitamin C is also essential for the absorption of iron.** Iron deficiencies are often caused by a lack of Vitamin C.

During stressful times, Vitamin C is quickly depleted because it is directly involved in the release of the stress hormones, epinephrine, cortizone and adrenaline produced by the adrenal glands. It is important in the production of thyroxin which is made by the thyroid gland and responsible for the regulation of basal metabolic rate (metabolism) as well as body temperature.

Symptoms of Vitamin C Depletion
Increased infection or colds, bleeding gums, anemia, cellulite, slow healing, easy bruising and fatigue are a few of the symptoms of Vitamin C depletion.

Supplementation
Most Americans are over-acidic and taking of large dosages of ascorbic acid or Vitamin C may contribute to further acidification of the stomach and kidneys. Ascorbic acid in large amounts raises urinal uric acid levels and may cause gout symptoms and even kidney stones. Most Vitamin C sup-

plements sold in pharmacies, health food stores and grocery stores **are** ascorbic acid. The label may read "Vitamin C with Rose Hips," "Vitamin C with Acerola Berries," or "Vitamin C with Bioflavonoids," but the Vitamin C is ascorbic acid! Within the human body, minerals like calcium, magnesium, sodium and potassium **buffer** acids. When a mineral combines with ascorbic acid, a complex called **ascorbate** is formed. The mineral has effectively buffered the free acid. Using a **calcium ascorbate supplement**, whereby the manufacturer has already combined the mineral calcium with Vitamin C, **has the benefits of calcium and the protective value of Vitamin C without the acid.** When taking Vitamin C in large doses (1,000 mg - 3,000 mg per day), the **ascorbated** form is the safest and best. The daily ingestion of Vitamin C is a wise and protective measure.

Food Sources of Vitamin C

Rose hips, acerola cherries, green peppers, apples, citrus and potatoes.

VITAMIN D

Vitamin D is fat-soluble and known as the "sunshine" vitamin.

Roles of Vitamin D

Vitamin D is essential to the proper absorption of calcium and phosphorous. It is also important in maintaining a stable nervous system, normal heart rate and blood clotting.

Caution

Vitamin D is found primarily in foods of animal origin, depending on how much exposure to the sun the animals have had. Eating 3 tablespoons of butter and an egg, provides only 65 of 400 I.U. of Vitamin D recommended. Because of the scarcity of Vitamin D in food, nature seems to suggest that exposure to sunlight is the best form of Vitamin D. Rickets, a deforming bone disease, is prevented by exposure to sunlight. In one study in England, it appeared Vitamin D obtained from the skin's exposure to sunlight was far superior to that which was obtained from oral ingestion. The more sunlight patients received, the more normal the calcium and phosphorous levels in the blood became. Bones also remained normal. Dietary Vitamin D had no bearing on the levels of calcium and phosphorous in the bloodstream. As sunlight strikes the skin, cholesterol (concentrated in skin) can be transformed into pre-vitamin D. After leaving the sunlight, wait approximately a half hour before showering in order to allow the changes necessary to produce the pre-vitamin D. **Showering immediately after sunbathing washes away cholesterol and other oils needed for Vitamin D absorption.** Vitamin D found in the skin is then absorbed into the bloodstream. Since Vitamin D is produced from cholesterol, as are the other major steroid hormones, some experts believe vitamin D is a hormone, not a vitamin. The structure of vitamin D is very similar to the chemical structure of other steroid hormones. If Vitamin D is a hormone, should food be fortified with a hormone? Rather than urging that Vitamin D, which is crucial to calcium utilization, be obtained by exposure to sunlight, "health educators" have chosen to supplement food with Vitamin D. Added Vitamin D to dairy products, beverages, baby foods, breakfast cereals, margarine, flour and animal feeds, results in a per-capita Vitamin D intake in the U.S. of 2,435 I.U. per day, or six times the recommended 400 I.U. per day.

Symptoms of Vitamin D Imbalances

Increased intake of Vitamin D is known to cause heart attacks in experimental animals, raise blood cholesterol levels, irritate blood vessel linings, promote joint diseases and arthritis, cause magnesium deficiencies and mental retardation in new born babies. Deficiencies of Vitamin D cause rickets. **I recommend that Vitamin D supplementation be removed from our food since we can safely obtain all the Vitamin D we need by spending thirty minutes in the sunshine.** Excess intake of Vitamin D in the diet causes calcium to deposit in the soft tissues which is known as calcification of the joints (arthritis), while exposure to the sunlight aids in the proper utilization of calcium, reducing arthritic symptoms.

Supplementation of Vitamin D

One-half hour of sunlight is optimum. Take fish oil capsules of A and D 10,000 I.U. per day **only** when exposure to sunlight is restricted.

Food Sources

Fish oils and sunflower seeds contain **natural** Vitamin D. Avoid foods with synthetic Vitamin D_2 added.

VITAMIN E

Vitamin E, a fat-soluble vitamin, is actually a complex called tocopherols. The forms of tocopherol are: alpha, beta, delta, epsilon, eta, gamma and zeta. Because of Vitamin E's ability to restore fertility in laboratory animals, it was given the name tocopherol (Greek word - Tokos) meaning "offspring." **Highest quality tocopherols are found in vegetable oils, grains, seeds, and nuts.**

Roles of Vitamin E

One well-known Vitamin E function is that of an **antioxidant.** An antioxidant prevents oxygen from converting unsaturated fatty acids, saturated fatty acids and Vitamin A into peroxides, which could be cancer producing. **By sparing oxygen from fats, Vitamin E helps supply the red blood cells with more pure oxygen which is carried to the heart and other organs.** Vitamin E seems to protect the lungs from air pollutant damage such as nitrogen dioxide and ozone. This important vitamin helps dilate blood vessels and thin blood, permitting adequate blood flow to and from the heart. Cellular aging specifically results from oxidation, and Vitamin E is helpful in retarding this process.

Symptoms of Vitamin E Deficiency

Possible symptoms of Vitamin E deficiency are inflammation of the pancreas, wasting muscles, abnormal fatty deposits in the muscles, faulty absorption of fat, infertility, sterility, anemia, edema, hormonal imbalances, kidney congestion, heart disease and cancer.

Vitamin E deficiency also causes red blood cells to rupture

and become more vulnerable to environmental pollutants and stresses.

Supplementation

Vitamin E's ability to bring precious oxygen to the cells, to protect red blood cells from destruction by food and environmental poisons and to aid the body in protecting itself against cancer-causing rancid fats, are reasons the Lazy Person is advised to seek its use.

Of the seven forms of tocopherols, **alpha-tocopherol** is the most active and powerful and has the greatest nutritional value. Take 100 I.U. to 200 I.U. of alpha-tocopherols with a fat containing meal for best absorption.

Food Sources of Vitamin E

Whole grains, nuts and seeds.

CONCLUSION

Most Americans are depleted in calcium, magnesium, potassium and Vitamins A, B, C and E due to their dietary patterns and urban lifestyles. Supplements give us that "edge" against processed foods, nutrient-poor soils and the stresses of a nuclear age. Since food supplements are concentrated sources of vitamins or minerals, deficiencies can be made up quickly within a few months or years. The Lazy Person wanting to save time, utilizes supplements. The following vitamins and minerals taken as directed, can be very beneficial.

Potassium (complexed) - 99 mg. or one tablet taken tiwce a day with meals

Vitamin E - 100-200 I.U. of alpha-tocopherols taken with a fat containing meal.

Vitamin C - 1,000-3,000 mg. of calcium ascorbates taken with or between meals

Vitamin A - 10,000-30,000 units of beta carotene taken with meals.

Calcium gluconate or chelate - 1,000 mg. before bedtime.

Magnesium Chelate - 500 mg. with breakfast or lunch

Vitamin D - one half hour in the sun - 10,000 I.U. of A and D fish oil capsules.

Vitamin B-Complex - 50 mg. (rice based) with meals.

DIRECTIONS FOR TAKING SUPPLEMENTS

1. Take supplements six days a week and rest on the seventh day.
2. Take supplements for three months, then discontinue for three months. One may create a dependency or even an immunity to supplements if taken too long. Resume supplements, if needed, after a three month rest.
3. Take supplements with meals unless otherwise advised by your nutritionist.

CAUTION

Although supplements are essential for replenishing vitamin and mineral deficiencies, taking multi-vitamin and multi-mineral supplements are not recommended. General assumptions may be made regarding vitamin and mineral deficiences caused by the Standard American Diet (S.A.D.), but every person's chemistry is different. **More specific recommendations should be made by your nutritionist after appropriate bio-chemical testing is completed.** Dietary and hereditary factors, marital status, sex, age, job stress and other variables make a multi-vitamin-mineral supplement designed for everyone, unrealistic. In fact, such supplements may even be dangerous. **Vitamins and minerals are not harmless, and taking unneeded supplements may cause the development of other deficiencies.**

Zinc has received the applause of many nutritionists, and for good reason. This mineral can be very healthful **if needed.** However, taking unneeded zinc depletes copper reserves, a mineral necessary for the utilization of iron and Vitamin C.

Except for the few recommendations in this chapter, do not use guess work with your body chemistry. Seek out a nutritionist!

IMPORTANT

Much of the public believes nutrition means taking vitamins. Because so many claims are made regarding vitamins' curative power, the United States has developed a multi-billion dollar vitamin industry. Although vitamins and minerals are helpful and necessary in a technological world, please remember that **vitamins are not food.** I hear so many say, "I don't eat right, but at least I take supplements!" Be aware that a supplement does what the word implies, it **supplements** a healthy diet. **Supplements do not and cannot replace a natural diet. It is not natural to take any pill.**

You cannot expect to be healthy living on coffee, donuts and supplements. Health does not work that way. There are no magic bullets to wellness. If you eat a nutritious diet of grains, seeds, nuts, fruit and vegetables and reduce your fat, meat, sugar and salt intake, the supplements you take will have a better absorption rate. A good diet improves digestion, absorption and assimilation of vital nutrients including supplements. **If you do not assimilate foods, you will not assimilate supplements.**

Man does not live by supplements alone!

*Most vitamins and minerals sold in pharmacies contain **coal tar** as a binder. This substance, which is used to pave streets, is cancer causing. Even some supplements sold in natural food stores have a coal tar base. Ask your local health food store or nutritionist which brands are safe.

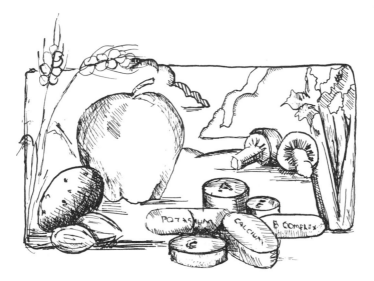

CHAPTER 6

WATER: ESSENTIAL FOR OPTIMUM HEALTH

"BETTER TO KEEP YOURSELF CLEAN AND BRIGHT: YOU ARE THE WINDOW THROUGH WHICH YOU MUST SEE THE WORLD." George Bernard Shaw

Next to air, water is the most essential substance our bodies need for maintaining optimum health. Water contains solutions to help regulate circulation, digestion and glandular functions, to name a few. In the digestive process, water is required by the salivary glands to mix with the food in order to swallow. It makes up the hydrochloric acid, pepsin and pancreatic enzymes essential for digestion of proteins, carbohydrates and fats, and carries nutrients to all the cells of the body. Water leaves the body as perspiration during exercise, removing some impurities. Water also cleanses bodily waste through the kidneys, eliminating three to six pints daily.

The average American uses 75 gallons of water within the home and an additional 100 gallons outside the home every day. Approximately 50% of the United States' water supply is used in the production of food. Growing a pound of wheat requires 85 gallons of water; growing a pound of rice, 500 gallons. Cattle and horses need and average of 8-15 gallons of water a day to survive! The quantity of water on planet earth is fixed, therefore water is reuseable and recyclable. **Every glass of water you drink contains water molecules that have existed since the earth was formed.**

We require 4-6 pints of fluid daily. This fluid is obtained not only from water, but also from various foods and drinks. **Too little water in our diets can cause the skin to shrink and wrinkle,** accounting for the nutritional statement that **sufficient water drinking helps maintain a beautiful complexion.**

We water our house plants, yet many of us don't drink adequate amounts of water to keep ourselves from drying out! The body is made up of 60% water and the brain 75% water.

Solubility of Water

One of the most distinctive and important properties of water is its **solubility.** Water has been called the **universal solvent** due to its capacity to dissolve most inorganic and some organic substances. As substances dissolve in water, particles break away from one another and are attracted to individual water molecules. The water molecule consists of one atom of oxygen and two atoms of hydrogen, forming H_2O. The extraordinary attraction of water for other substances makes it somewhat like a bar magnet. In its chemical composition the top-heavy hydrogen atoms are positively charged and the oxygen atom at the bottom is negatively charged.

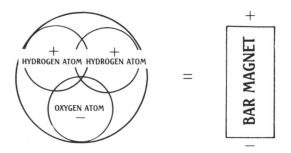

The natural capacity for water to attract and dissolve a variety of substances makes it difficult to find absolutely pure water. As a mountain stream continues its journey down the mountain, it comes in contact with metals, wastematter, gases and many other pollutants. Since water is naturally contaminated, nature provides a purification process to rid water of its impurities. Recycling of the water on earth is done by a gigantic distiller powered by the sun. Water from the earth is evaporated into the atmosphere (leaving impurities behind), and as the water vapor cools, it condenses back into water. The water falls back to earth as rain, snow or other precipitations. Rainwater would be the purest distilled water to drink if not for its solubility. As water falls through the air, pollutants, chemicals and bacteria are attracted which help to recontaminate the water. Acid rain is an example of this contamination process.

Besides natural pollutants which water attracts, other dangerous pollutants accumulate in water on earth. Bacterial contamination from animals and livestock, industrial pollutants (chemicals) and agricultural pollutants such as pesticides, herbicides and fungicides are a few of these pollutants. Water treatment plants throughout our nation "purify" this contaminated water by adding chemicals such as floride, chlorine, copper sulfate and aluminum sulfate to disinfect and deodorize. Other chemicals remove minerals that cause "hardness."

Some chemicals used in water treatment are considered controversial and a form of contamination themselves. Chlorine, used to disinfect the water by killing bacteria, could be just as effective in killing the "friendly bacteria" of your digestive tract. The addition of copper and aluminum sulfates could cause accumulation of these chemicals in your body over time. Alzheimer's Disease, found in growing numbers of the elderly, affects the brain. Those with this condition can become totally disoriented and lose their memory. Research indicates that accumulations of aluminum in the brain **could be the cause** of Alzheimer's Disease. Could aluminum in city water supplies be the culprit? Some authorities consider fluoridation of public drinking water another form of contamination. Studies in the 1950's concluded that natural-occurring calcium fluoride in some water supplies reduced tooth decay. The fluoride added to our drinking water today **is not** naturally occurring calcium fluoride; instead it is **sodium** fluoride. Besides getting more **sodium** from drinking tap water (see Chapter Seven) some experts feel sodium fluoride can be cancer producing.

Most argue that the small amounts of these chemical additives, one or two parts per million, can do no harm. The immediate danger of these chemicals to human health is not in question. What is in question is the cumulative effect. Could using "safe levels" of toxic chemicals for twenty or thirty years collect within organs and tissues producing such diseases as Alzheimer's or cancer? Only time and research will give us the answers. **The Lazy Person, realizing the potential danger of chemicalized water, does not wait until "enough" scientific proof is gathered.**

Another question concerning contamination of city water systems concerns the "purified" water which leaves the water treatment plant. Consider the underground pipes that deliver the water to our homes, as well as the plumbing inside our homes. Worn or outdated water pipes permit soil pollutants to enter pipelines. Water's solubility, as discussed earlier in the chapter, allows the collection of metals such as iron, copper, lead and cadmium. Such toxic metals may be present in your underground pipelines.

Minerals In Water

Hard water deposits found in tea kettles, sink faucets and drains are caused by such inorganic minerals as calcium, magnesium, sodium and iron. Some researchers believe that the accumulation of such inorganic minerals over time contributes to the following problems: arthritis, rheumatism, hardening of the arteries and kidney failure. Placing tap water in a standard iron causes steel corrosion which is why directions suggest **distilled water only.** If minerals and chemicals present in tap water can eat away steel, what do you suppose they can do to human flesh?

Authorities argue that minerals in water help nourish the body. One should receive nutrients from food, not water. Pure water is primarily needed to cleanse the body, particularly the kidneys, of toxins and poisons such as drugs, pesticides, herbicides, antibiotics, and air pollutants. Due to water's solubility and magnetic properties, it cleanses these body pollutants through the kidneys. Your kidneys then filter harmful waste products and cellular debris from metabolism into the urine, keeping your blood pure. When a kidney cannot properly function, valuable protein and minerals like potassium, calcium, magnesium, and zinc are filtered into the urine instead of into the bloodstream. Furthermore, if a kidney's delicate filtration system malfunctions, blood cannot be purified, which may result in tissue poisoning. Additionally, kidney failure problems include: high blood pressure, water retention, great thirst, cramping and fatigue. Poor kidney functions may also result in accumulations of calcium, magnesium and oxalic acid in the kidneys, causing **stones.**

However, water drinking is essential in order to assist your kidneys to eliminate cellular metabolism and toxic waste products resulting from a modern industrial society. The Lazy Person looks for an alternative solution to obtaining the pure water he needs.

WHAT WATER IS BEST?

Since rainwater is the purest water we can drink, it would be our first choice if it were not for the air pollutants it collects. Experts who suggest distilled water is unnatural, forget that distillation is the process by which all water is purified and returned to the earth.

Next to distilled rain water, **steam distilled water,** is the purest water available. Di-ionized water purified by electrical current is not recommended. I recommend drinking steam distilled water for 3-6 months in order to detoxify the body and kidneys of poisons. **Just as rain water falling through the atmosphere acts like a magnet to attract pollutants, steam distilled water attracts the poisons and carries them into the urine via the kidneys.**

Recommendation

Drink 1 oz. of water for every 2 pounds of body weight. **Example:** If you weigh 130 lbs. - drink 65 oz. of water or 8 cups per day.

After an initial cleansing period of 3 to 6 months, replace distilled water with "low sodium" spring water obtained from a water company. Many bottled water companies deliver distilled and spring water to your home. Supermarkets also carry bottled water.

Caution

Water is very hot after the distillation process, and if poured immediately into plastic bottles, it can attract the plastic. If water tastes plastic after opening, return it. **Use glass bottles whenever possible.**

When To Drink Water

Few people today have good digestion; stomach bloating, gas and acid buildup are commonplace. Excess salt in the diet causes many Americans to drink with their meals. The American habit of "flushing" food down causes many of these gastric disturbances. One of the fundamental rules of good digestion is: **Don't drink water or other liquids with meals. Water dilutes and weakens the digestive juices of the stomach. Drink water 30 minutes before or 30 minutes after main meals and watch your digestion improve!**

Although pure water is essential to the health of the body, gluttony with water is as harmful as gluttony with food. **Waiting until you are starved before eating or very thirsty before drinking leads to gluttony and is not the Lazy Person's way.** Your kidneys are only slightly larger than your ears, and can be overworked by excessive water drinking. One cup (8 oz.) of water every hour or two is adequate to regulate the crucial role of your kidneys.

Of all the blood pumped out of the heart (8,000 quarts a day), one fifth (20%), nearly 1,700 quarts, passes to the kidneys for the purpose of making one to two quarts of urine each day. Drinking sufficient quantities of pure water daily helps this remarkable organ (kidneys) filter wastes from the blood and regulates the volume and composition of fluids and nutrients constituting the internal environment of your body.

Conclusion

We live in both an external environment, and an internal liquid environment which preserves and feeds our organs, tissues and cells. **The greatest thirst quencher of all time is cool, clear, clean water.** Developing the positive habit of drinking water will provide the Lazy Person with part of the health insurance needed to live an energetic life. Let's drink to that!

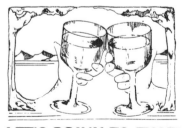

LET'S DRINK TO THAT!

CHAPTER 7

SALT: SHAKE THE HABIT

"THE WORST BOSS TO HAVE IS A BAD HABIT."

Most Americans are aware of only one kind of salt - table salt (sodium chloride). However, many other salts play key roles in the digestive process. Without sodium bicarbonate (a buffer), strong acids produced by the stomach could burn holes along your digestive tract. Sodium and potassium salts are called electrolytes, and transmit electrical currents throughout the nervous system. Potassium salts are important to the activities of the brain and the contraction of muscles, especially the heart. Potassium is also a very important nutrient for heart and brain cells. These are a few of the numerous salts needed by your body.

Even though salt is essential to your system, in excess it can be very dangerous. Adults need approximately 400 mg., or 1/5 of a teaspoon of salt daily to maintain optimum health and internal balance. The average American adult consumes 2 to 2 1/2 teaspoons of salt every day; more than 10 times the bodily requirement. **Salt excess in the American diet is derived from table salt and/or sea salt.** Both **table salt** and **sea salt** are processed salts and extremely high in sodium chloride (90%-99%). **The overconsumption of sodium chloride depletes your body of needed potassium.** Without enough potassium, symptoms such as loss of memory, mental confusion, heart palpitations and water retention may be experienced. **Women seem to be very sensitive to potassium loss and often experience swelling and weight gain. (See Chapter Five).** Your kidneys are responsible for eliminating water and excess salt from your body. The kidneys filter all the sodium and potassium out of the bloodstream, and with great precision, return the exact amount needed to the blood. **Excessive amounts of salt overwork the kidneys, contributing to water retention** and **potassium loss.** Such excess load on the kidneys will damage their delicate filtration system. Dark circles and puffiness under the eyes are signs of overworked kidneys.

The connection between overconsumption of **salt** and **hypertension is as clear as the line between high cholesterol and heart disease.** More than 60 million Americans suffer from hypertension, and nearly one half of the population over the age of 65 is affected by the conditon. Too much salt can reduce the diameter of your arteries leading to high blood pressure. If you have ever seen meat cured by salt, you know that the salt pulls the water and blood out of the mean (like beef jerky). **Excess salt in the bloodstream will pull the fluid out of an artery causing it to constrict, or become smaller.** In other words, the smaller the diameter of the artery, the higher the blood pressure.

The popular belief that fats, such as cholesterol, accumulate on the arterial walls causing them to narrow, is actually the second step in arteriosclerosis. The first step to this disease is actually excess salt in the blood which constricts arteries and produces fat deposits.

High blood pressure, or hypertension, is the most significant factor influencing both strokes and heart attacks in the United States, Japan and other industrialized countries. The Japanese probably consume more salt than any other culture in the world. Their diet includes nearly 3 teaspoons of salt each day, consumed in foods such as fish, pickled vegetables and soy seasoned rice (1,029 mg. per tablespoon). Japan leads the world in hypertension, and it comes as no surprise that their leading cause of death is strokes. In the United States, approximately 550,000 strokes occur annually, resulting in an estimated 162,000 deaths, while 1,250,000 heart attacks result in 550,000 deaths. **In simpler cultures** like Hunza, Abkhazia (Russia) and Vilcabambas (Equador), as well as the tribes of New Guinea, the Amazon Basin, the highlands of Malaysia, and rural Uganda, **little or no salt is eaten and hypertension does not exist.** The blood pressure of these healthy cultures does not rise with age as it does in the salt-loving nations like the United States and Japan. **When salt is added to the diet of an otherwise low-salt culture, blood pressure elevates.** Hundreds of test results have shown the cause-effect relationship between salt intake and hypertension strokes and heart attacks.

The latest research on sodium strongly suggests that high sodium primes your brain to be hypersensitive to stress. Salt increases the number of brain-cell receptors for norepinephrine, the nervous system hormone that prepares the body for "fight or flight" in dangerous situations. Norepinephrine sends messages from the brain to the heart (heart pumps faster), the digestive system (all organs stop digestion), and the blood vessels (vessels constrict). With more norepinephrine produced because of salt overconsumption, a person becomes increasingly nervous and edgy.

Excess salts can also accumulate in the body due to protein overconsumption. We all know we need protein in our diet, but what we don't know is that protein can become salt if eaten in excess. Protein breaks down into amino acids, and amino acids are dibasic. An amino acid in contact with a base element gives up two hydrogen atoms and becomes salt. Overconsumption of protein leads to a buildup of these unneeded salts in the ligaments, tendons, cartilage and connective tissues of the arteries and veins. Such salt buildup produces inflexible joints, brittle tendons and weak cartilage.

WHAT CAN A LAZY PERSON DO TO REDUCE SALT INTAKE?

1. **One half of all salt that Americans eat is added during processing.** Stop, or at least limit, intake of processed and packaged foods. Eliminate canned foods from your diet, and replace them with frozen and fresh alternatives. Salt (sodium chloride) is not the only source of sodium in processed food. Other common types of sodium used are: Monosodium glutamate, sodium nitrate, sodium benzoate, disodium phosphate, baking soda and baking powder. If you must buy processed foods, read the labels carefully. **Choose those foods that are labeled "low sodium" or "salt free".** Limit all soft drinks. Carbonated drinks contain bicarbonate of soda (sodium bicarbonate). Replace pop and diet pop with unsweetened fruit juices, unsalted vegetable juices and **bottled water** (the best thirst quencher of all). Most tap water contains too much sodium to be a healthy alternative (see Chapter Six).

Instead of high sodium dairy products, use unsalted butter and low sodium cheese. **Plain, unsweetened yogurt contains no added salt and is a healthier alternative to cheese.**

Eat raw, unsalted nuts like almonds, hazelnuts and pecans. Peanuts are highly acidic and difficult to digest (peanuts are actually legumes - part of the pea family, and are not nuts). Replace peanut butter with almond butter, which is alkaline forming and easy to digest.

Seafoods, like clams, shrimp, scallops, crab and lobster are all high in salt content. They may be replaced with fish like bass, salmon, trout, red snapper and cod. For a complete fish list, see Chapter 2.

A good rule of thumb to remember: **THE MORE PROCESS-ED A FOOD, THE HIGHER THE SALT CONTENT.**

HIDDEN SALT

APPLE 2mg salt	APPLESAUCE 1 cup 6mg salt	APPLE PIE 1/8 frozen 208mg salt
BUTTER 1 T unsalted 2mg salt	BUTTER 1 T salted 16mg salt	MARGARINE 1 T 140mg salt
CHICKEN 1/2 breast 69mg salt	CHICKEN PIE Frozen 907mg salt	CHICKEN Fast Food 2,243mg salt
CORN 1mg salt	FLAKES 1 c 256mg salt	CANNED 1 c 384mg salt
CUCUMBER 7 slices 2mg salt	CUCUMBER w/dressing 234mg salt	DILL PICKLE 928mg salt
GRAPES 10 seedless 1mg salt	GRAPE JELLY 1 T 3mg salt	WHITE WINE 4 oz domestic 19mg salt
LEMON 1mg salt	SOY SAUCE 1 T 1,029mg salt	SALT 1 T 1,938mg salt
MILK 1 c 122mg salt	DRY MILK 1/2 c 322mg salt	COTTAGE CHEESE 4 oz 457mg salt
POTATO 5mg salt	CHIPS 10 200mg salt	INSTANT 1 c 485mg salt
TOMATO 14mg salt	SOUP 1 c 932mg salt	SAUCE 1 c 1,498mg salt
TUNA 3 oz 50mg salt	TUNA 3 oz canned 384mg salt	TUNA PIE Frozen 715mg salt
WATER 8 oz tap 12mg salt	CLUB SODA 8 oz 39mg salt	ANTACID in water 564mg salt

Source: U.S. Department of Agriculture Handbook #8.

2. One quarter of all the salt we consume is added during cooking or at the dinner table. Empty your salt shakers! Fill them with another flavoring. Eliminating salt doesn't mean eliminating flavor. Instead, season your food with herbs and spices like garlic, onions, dill, cayenne and curry (to name but a few). These spices come in powder form and are great flavor enhancers. Try some ginger root, lemon, lime, thyme, basil, and tumeric to flavor soups, casseroles and meat dishes.

Although some salt substitutes appear to reduce salt content, they may have just replaced the sodium chloride with another salt like potassium chloride. Such substitutes can upset your sodium and potassium chemical balance and are not recommended. A few salt alternatives derived from dried vegetables having the correct sodium-potassium balance are:

1. **Quick Sip** - a substitute for soy sauce - made by Jensen.

2. **Vegetable Broth Seasoning** - a salt like powder seasoning made by Jensen.

3. **Vegit** - a herb based powder seasoning made by Hauser.

4. **Sea Vegetation** - made by Wachters

These products, as well as other fine salt substitutes, can be purchased in supermarket health food sections or natural food stores.

3. One quarter of all the salt we consume occurs naturally in food.

Unlike table salt or sea salt which are high in sodium and almost totally devoid of potassium, natural sodium present in fresh, unprocessed foods is balanced with potassium. That's the way mother nature intended it! **There is enough natural salt in a wholesome diet of grains, seeds, nuts, vegetables and fruits to satisfy the adult daily sodium requirement (400 mg.)** A half of a cup of cooked brown rice, for instance, contains 282 mg. of natural sodium.

CONCLUSION

Although sodium is essential for the proper metabolic functions, excess salt consumption irritates the nervous system, increases the blood pressure and the heart beat. Excess salt also robs the body of calcium and B-complex vitamins. Retention of salt in the tissues leaves a person water logged and bloated.

Eliminating salt from your diet improves circulation (no more cold hands and feet), eliminates extra water weight (no more puffy eyes and swollen hands), and significantly reduces your chances of developng heart disease, the number one killer in the United States. **THE LAZY PERSON REALIZES THAT YOU DON'T "CATCH" DISEASE, YOU EAT IT AND YOU DRINK IT.** The Lazy Person is interested in results. Therefore, I suggest giving up table salt for 3 months and experiencing the natural flavor of foods. We can receive all the sodium our bodies require from a wholesome diet of grains, seeds, nuts, vegetables and fruits. Since reduction of salt intake poses no risk to your health, the Lazy Person would be wise to say, "When it comes to salt, **SHAKE THE HABIT!!**"

CHAPTER 8

SUGAR: FRIEND OR FOE

"IT IS A WISE MAN WHO KNOWS THE COMPANY TO KEEP AWAY FROM."

The human brain and most human body functions depend on glucose, or sugar, for energy (see Chapter Three). Some nutritionists argue that all sugar ends up as glucose in the bloodstream making it insignificant what sort of sugar a person chooses to eat. Although natural and processed sugars do eventually break down into glucose, **the speed at which the sugar enters the bloodstream is crucial.** Complex sugars, such as those in grains and fruits, digest slowly causing no drastic elevation in blood sugar levels. However, concentrated or simple sugars enter the blood stream very quickly due to their elementary molecular structure (mono and disaccarhides). Simple sugars include white sugar, brown sugar, honey, molasses, maple syrup and fructose (in refined form). Since simple sugars enter the bloodstreem rapidly, quick energy lifts are experienced. If too much sugar reaches the blood too quickly, the amount of oxygen transported by the blood slows down, and the brain and body extremities do not receive enough oxygen. **White sugar robs your cells of needed oxygen.**

The pancreas helps maintain the proper blood sugar level through secretion of a hormone called **insulin.** This organ **reduces** sugar levels in the blood by secreting insulin which carries extra sugar to the liver where it is converted into glycogen. Glycogen is stored in the liver and muscles and released when your energy or blood sugar is low. With the aid of the adrenal glands, glycogen is then converted back into glucose. The adrenal glands can secrete a hormone called epinephrine or adrenaline, which when combined with stored glycogen, produces glucose to raise blood sugar levels. Your body has the capacity to either lower blood sugar (insulin) or raise blood sugar (glycogen and adrenaline) as needed.

The average American eats 120 to 150 pounds of refined white sugar a year. Our pancreas was not designed to constantly secrete large amounts of insulin in order to reduce high levels of processed white sugar. **If your pancreas is forced to overproduce insulin for an extended period of time (20-30 years), you run the risk of damaging the insulin producing mechanism.** Diabetes is a condition where too little insulin is produced and sugar levels in the blood remain high. Amputation of arms and legs as well as blindness due to a lack of adequate oxygen (remember excess sugar blocks oxygen transportation) are some tragic results of Diabetes. Eight out of every ten cases of diabetes in the U.S. are Type II, or the adult-onset type. **A diabetic (high blood sugar) condition is created by eating refined white sugar.** According to the book, **Sugar Blues,** the first step leading to diabetes is low blood sugar as a result of long-time insulin overproduction. **Your pancreas will exhaust itself after years of refined sugar intake, causing diabetes.**

If you have symptoms such as depression, nervousness, irritability, loss of memory, sudden fatigue, dizziness, headaches, sweet cravings, protein cravings, blurred vision or mental confusion, it could mean you have low blood sugar, or worse, hypoglycemia.

Most people experience an increase in energy after eating a candy bar or other sugar product, only to feel an energy crash approximately 20 minutes later. The secretion of a large amount of insulin by your pancreas in order to quickly lower the blood sugar causes this low energy response. Mood swings, depression and fatigue are common during this crash period.

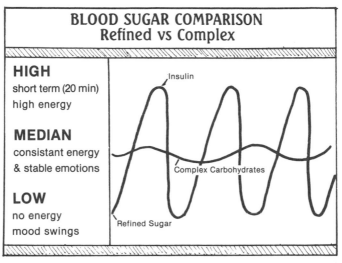

BLOOD SUGAR COMPARISON
Refined vs Complex

HIGH
short term (20 min)
high energy

MEDIAN
consistant energy
& stable emotions

LOW
no energy
mood swings

Insulin

Complex Carbohydrates

Refined Sugar

Although most Americans refrain from adding refined sugar to foods, sugar is in everything.

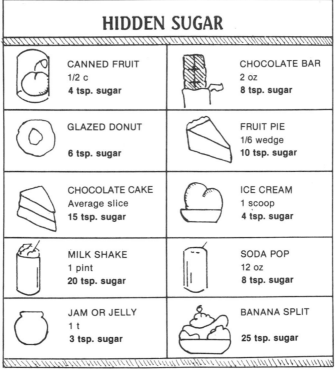

HIDDEN SUGAR

CANNED FRUIT 1/2 c **4 tsp. sugar**		CHOCOLATE BAR 2 oz **8 tsp. sugar**	
GLAZED DONUT **6 tsp. sugar**		FRUIT PIE 1/6 wedge **10 tsp. sugar**	
CHOCOLATE CAKE Average slice **15 tsp. sugar**		ICE CREAM 1 scoop **4 tsp. sugar**	
MILK SHAKE 1 pint **20 tsp. sugar**		SODA POP 12 oz **8 tsp. sugar**	
JAM OR JELLY 1 t **3 tsp. sugar**		BANANA SPLIT **25 tsp. sugar**	

Source: Loma Linda University.

Besides finding refined sugar in pies, cakes, candies and ice ceam, we find it added to many other foods. Sugar constitutes more than one third of the ingredients in commercial salad dressing, ketchups and boxed cereals. It is added to soups, gravies, hot dogs, and luncheon meats. **Sugar goes by many aliases: corn syrup or corn sweetener, fructose, dextrose, sucrose, raw sugar and brown sugar.** Some food labels list two or three different sweeteners in their ingredients. Even though these sugars do not appear as the number one or two ingredient, the sum of the sugars are greater than any other ingredient.

Refined white sugar contains almost no vitamins or minerals and has 385 calories per 100 grams (3 1/2 ounces). Honey has only traces of vitamins and minerals and 305 calories per 100 gram portion. Neither refined sugar nor honey are good for blood sugar maintenance or weight control. Sugar alcohols or substitutes such as xylitol, mannitol and sorbitol, which many eat for weight loss, also have many calories.

Aspartame, commonly known as NutraSweet, is approximately 180 times sweeter than sugar and has very few calories. Aspartame is composed of two amino acids, phenylalanine and aspartic acid. With heat and time, aspartame breaks down into methyl alcohol or wood alcohol. Methyl alcohol is a well-known poison. **Ninety-five percent of aspartame becomes formaldehyde in the body, a cancer-producing agent.** Artificial sweeteners, such as cyclamates and sacchrin, have been banned because of the cancers they caused in laboratory animals. We do not know what a "safe level" of methyl alcohol is, or if small amounts of this toxic substance ingested over many years will produce cancers in humans. Other critics remind us of studies indicating that phenylalanine could impair brain development in fetuses of women who are carriers of PKU (phenylketonuria), an inherited metabolic disease. Since most pregnant women are not likely to know whether they are carriers of PKU or not, critics recommend that all pregnant women avoid using aspartame. The other amino acid, aspartic acid, is absorbed quickly by the brain, and tests on laboratory animals suggest that high quantities of this amino acid also cause brain damage. Common Cause, a Washington D.C. based consumer group is challenging the approval of NutraSweet (aspartame) by the Food and Drug Administration. The author agrees with Common Cause that evidence supporting aspartame's safety to public health is inconclusive for F.D.A. approval.

The Lazy Person would not subject his body to potentially harmful effects of an additive like NutraSweet, and would have to admit that there still is **no safe artificial sweetener available.**

REFINED SUGAR IS A THIEF

All sugar eaten, whether natural or refined, requires B-complex vitamins, calcium and magnesium to aid in digestion. Natural carbohydrates, such as grains and fruits, contain enough of these nutrients to assist the body in their own digestion. Refining sugar (white or brown) removes these, and many other precious vitamins and minerals. **B-complex is taken from the nervous system and calcium and magnesium from the bones and teeth to digest refined sugars.** Consequently, refined sugar "rips you off" of these needed nutrients resulting in "raw" nerves.

According to statistics, most of us can expect to have some form of osteoporosis, or arthritis in our lifetime. Osteoporosis is the thinning of bones or removal of calcium from the bones. **One of the leading causes of osteoporosis is the use of refined sugar, which forces the body to use up its own calcium and magnesium storage.** As calcium and magnesium are removed from the bones, they end up in the soft tissues of the body, including the hair and the joints. This accumulation of calcium in the joints is commonly referred to as arthritis. Approximately 75% of men and women over 60 have some form of osteoporosis or arthritis. **Is it old age which causes these degenerative conditions, or the consumption of the thief called refined sugar?**

CONCLUSION

The Select Committee on Nutrition and Human Needs, United States Senate, made an exhaustive study of

Americans' eating patterns. In a government document entitled "Dietary Goals for the United States," the fifth recommendation suggests Americans should reduce consumption of refined sugars by 45% and increase the complex carbohydrates (grains, seeds, nuts, vegetables and fruit) to 60%. I would like to stress that grains are good sources of B-complex, calcium, and magnesium and are full of natural glucose, which is assimilated over several hours.

Harmful effects of eating refined or simple sugars are the development of degenerative diseases such as diabetes, hypoglycemia, osteoporosis and arthritis. **Complex carbohydrates, not refined sugar, are the time-released sugars the brain and cells need to function optimally.** As long as Americans do not eat complex carbohydrates in their diets, they will crave refined sugars. **The solution to breaking the sugar habit is to replace simple sugars with complex ones.** Start including grains like millet, buckwheat, brown rice, and oats in your diet every day, and your cravings for candy bars, pop, and junk foods will decrease. **SAYING "NO" TO SUGAR IS NOT SUFFICIENT TO MAINTAIN GOOD HEALTH: YOU MUST SAY "YES" TO GRAINS.**

CHAPTER 9

ALLERGIES: MODERN DAY PLAGUE

"WHEN WE'RE THROUGH CHANGING - WE'RE THROUGH!"
Paul H. Dunn

Food allergies have become a major problem for many Americans. The dictionary definition of an allergy is "a heightened sensitivity to a substance." These "substances" are called **allergens** and provoke allergic reactions. Some allergic reactions are mild and subtle such as slight headaches, fatigue, anxiety, depression, respiratory infections, light headedness and weight gain. A sensitivity to a food often inflames the tissues of the body, adding extra pounds due to fluid retention. **Consequently, no matter how little an allergic person eats, he may not lose weight.**

An allergy irritates the nervous system. **Histamine,** produced by the cells, helps the nerve messages jump from one nerve ending to the next, and in an allergic response, cells produce excess histamine. Cells then discharge excess histamine through weaker cell membranes, irritating tissue and dilating or expanding blood vessels. Fluids that leak from both tissues and blood vessels cause the swelling and inflammation often associated with allergies. **Inflammation is a natural response to an allergen.** Many allergic people take anti-histamines to combat and reduce the inflammation. Leakage of fluids within an inflamed area permit white blood cells (soldiers in the body who defend against infection) easy entry to the allergen. The inflammation also blocks (walls off) the allergen and keeps it from spreading to the rest of your body.

In Dr. Paavo Airola's classic, **EVERYWOMAN'S BOOK,** he states that **babies do not have the enzymes necessary to digest any other food but mother's milk until six to eight months.** Healthy cultures breast feed their young for at least 6 months to 2 years before introducing other foods. Many mothers introduce other foods to their babies as early as six weeks. The first food given to infants are cow's milk, pablum, cream of wheat and orange juice. **To a newborn, these undigestible foods are "foreign invaders", similar to viruses or germs.** Consequently, infants manufacture specific antibodies to fight these foods. As adults, we continue to produce these antibodies in order to fight the foreign invaders, milk, wheat, and oranges. Statistics indicate that the primary allergic foods in the United States are wheat, milk and citrus.

According to pioneer nutritionist, Dr. Bernard Jensen, 29% of all the food we consume in the United States is wheat based and 25% is milk based (milk, cheese, cottage cheese and butter). Since more than half the food we eat is derived from only two sources, it is no wonder that many of us continue to experience sensitivities to these foods. Dr. Jensen describes allergies by saying we have become **"wheat logged", "milk logged"** and **"citrus logged."**

COW'S MILK

Milk is a food which produces excess mucus, congesting the lungs and making breathing difficult. Some allergic symptoms that infants develop include asthma, nasal congestion, skin rashes and various chest infections. **In addition, other less noticeable symptoms are irritability and fatigue.**

There are two types of milk allergies: 1) **Lactase deficiency** - those that cannot digest the lactose in milk. This allergy causes gas, bloating, cramps, mucus buildup, constipation and/or diarrhea. 2) **Casein sensitivity** - those allergic to the protein, casein, contained in cow's milk. This allergy causes similar disturbances to those of lactase deficiency. **Adults of African or Oriental descent are most often lactase deficient.** This condition is less common in the United States, where many people are of northern European ancestry. **Most Americans experience a casein intolerance because babies are given cow's milk instead of being breast fed.**

The principal protein in cow's milk is casein, which enables the cow to grow into a 1,000 pound animal. **When fed to an infant, approximately 50% or more of the casein is not digested.** Partially digested protein (casein) in the bloodstream irritates all the tissues of the body, increasing sensitivities to other allergens. **Although cow's milk is a good source of calcium, many humans do not have the ability to absorb it properly.**

On the other hand, the primary protein in mother's milk is **lactoalbumin,** which is easily digested by babies. The calcium in mother's milk is completely digested and utilized by the infant. **Mother's milk, not cow's milk, is the perfect food for infants.**

This intolerance to cow's milk continues throughout adulthood. Milk, one of the leading allergy producers, is a no-no for the Lazy Person who wants to avoid allergies.

Healthy cultures drink very little milk, and when they do, it is usually goat milk which is nutritionally similar to mother's milk. Additionally, healthy cultures eat very little cheese. Besides cheese having a high cholesterol and high sodium content, it is also extremely binding (constipating). **I call cheese "solidified mucus."** Cheese contributes to both constipation and allergy symptoms. Healthy cultures prefer clabbered or soured milk products to milk or cheese. Plain yogurt, a cultured dairy product, is made by fermenting milk with two kinds of bacteria, **lactobacillus bulgaricus** and **streptococcus thermophilus.** These organisms create lactase, which becomes active in the small intestine (the heat within the small intestine assist this process.) Lactase breaks down milk sugar (lactose) which is then easily absorbed into the bloodstream. **Yogurt digests itself, unlike milk or cheese, and enhances the "friendly bacteria" of the large intestine (colon), which improves elimination.** Studies demonstrate that people absorb lactose in yogurt about 66% better than the equivalent amount of lactose in milk. **I recommend plain, unsweetened yogurt which can be purchased in any grocery or health food store.** Yogurt bacteria is damaged or destroyed in a few days when mixed with sugar, fructose, or honey. Buying plain yogurt, or better still, making your own and adding apple juice concentrate or other fruit concentrates and/or fruit such as bananas, strawberries and peaches, insures the active bacteria. Yogurt and kefir are the easiest to digest and will not cause allergic responses in most milk-allergic people.

WHEAT

Some healthy cultures do eat whole, cooked wheat berries (cooked like rice) and whole wheat flour tortillas. But these foods are eaten **along with** other grains like beans, corn, rice or lentils and not exclusively. However, cultures do not refine the wheat as we do in the United States.

Wheat is very high in gluten, a protein substance. Remember making paper mache glue as children? What did we make this glue out of? White flour, (refined wheat), and water. The stickiness of the glue results from gluten (glue-ton). Wheat is the highest of all grains in gluten content. This sticky gluten creates mucus that can clog the bronchial tubes and lungs.* Those with severe wheat allergies know what I'm saying about gluten, and the rest of you can try an experiment. Eliminate wheat from your diet for the next three months, then begin eating it again. Notice any of the symptoms mentioned earlier, as well as actual cold symptoms? **REMEMBER THAT YOU ARE YOUR OWN EXPERIMENTAL LABORATORY. YOU CAN SPEND AS MUCH OR LITTLE TIME AS YOU WISH WORKING IN THAT LABORATORY.**

How many times have you known someone who just couldn't lose weight though they ate very little. Many of my clients especially women, drop those extra pounds as soon as they eliminate wheat from their diets.

You may wonder what you can use in place of wheat since it is eaten so much in our culture. I recommend rice flour because it is gluten-free, delicious and lower in calories. Local supermarkets and health food stores carry rice flour as well as oat, soy, buckwheat and rye flour.**

*   Whole wheat and white flour create the same allergy response.

**   See wheat-free cookbooks listed in back of book.

ORANGES

Oranges are the third most allergy producing food in the United States. Because they are usually picked green, sugars and citric acid are not permitted to mature properly. **Green citric acid** is very acid forming and this strong acid could damage both the stomach and the kidneys.

Oranges are also high in **alanine,** an amino acid which can deplete **lysine,** another amino acid. **Lysine seems to be con-ected with the immune or infection fighting mechanism of our bodies.** Viruses such as cold sores (fever blisters) and genital herpes, improve when large doses of lysine (2,000-4,000 mg. a day) are administered. Perhaps the overuse of oranges and orange juice since **early** childhood has actual-ly reduced our resistance to viruses despite the Vitamin C content. **Many people are sensitive to citrus, especially oranges, and do not realize it.**

As long as the fiber of the fruit is included (whole fruit), it will digest slowly (approximately 80 minutes), releasing sugar into the bloodstream at an acceptable and safe rate (see Chapters Three and Eight). Although oranges are wonderful energy foods, using the juice of oranges can raise the blood sugar too quickly (in a few minutes) forcing the pancreas to overwork.

Juices such as apple, pineapple and carrot, are excellent sources of naturally-occuring sugar and minerals and are best taken by diluting them with water (one half water to one half juice). Orange and grape juice **is not** recommended for people with low blood sugar or hypoglycemic symptoms. **WHENEVER POSSIBLE, EAT THE WHOLE FRUIT RATHER THAN THE JUICE.**

RESISTANCE

I recommend that most Americans remove wheat, milk, and citrus from their diets in order to regain and rebuild their resistance. **Health is a matter of resistance.** If six people worked in an office and one of them had a cold, what do you suppose would happen? Some would "catch" the cold and some would not. Why? All were breathing the cold germs, so the germs aren't the cause of the cold. The reason some got a cold and some didn't was — **Resistance. The stonger your im-munity to infection, the healthier you feel.** When allergy testing is given to people with low resistance, they will be "allergic" to many foods, including wholesome ones. **Any food can be a potential enemy or stress to someone with low immunity.** Tiredness and fatigue are intial signs of lowered resistance. The removal of wheat, milk and citrus aids your body in raising resistance and lowering over-sensitivity. Try it for three months and see! After strength is regained, adding a small percentage of these substances won't harm you.

ADRENAL SUPPORT

The adrenal glands are part of your body's immune system and sit on top of your kidneys. Cortisone, a drug given to fight infections or allergies, can be produced naturally by the adrenal glands. Adrenaline, given to people during asthma attacks, can also be naturally produced by the adrenal glands. Adrenaline prevents inflammation. It is produced when your body is under attack. When the adrenals are functioning properly, your body can easily handle minor invaders like pollen. **However, when adrenal glands are weak, allergens cannot be controlled and inflammation results.**

Dr. Hans Seyle, a Nobel prize-winning biologist, injected a strong allergen into rats. Rats with over-active adrenals had no reaction to the allergen, rats with normal adrenals had minor allergic reactions and rats with removed adrenals hemorrhaged, went into allergic shock and died within hours.

The importance of the adrenals in preventing allergies is well known today. Besides eliminating wheat, milk and citrus from the diet in order to increase resistance, **several supplements are very effective for strengthening the adrenal glands. Panthothenic acid,** or B_5, a key nutrient for the adrenal glands, provides fast relief from allergies. In extreme attacks, chew a 100 mg. tablet every hour until the attack subsides. **Calcium** is a natural antibiotic and also helps fight infection and allergy. **Hydrochloric acid,** necessary for the stomach to absorb calcium, is often depleted in allergic persons. **Vitamin C ascorbate** is another key nutrient which supports the adrenal glands. And **Vitamin E** is a natural antihistamine which helps block inflammatory responses. Vitamin E also helps T-cell production which is very important to the immune defense system of the body. Complete **B-complex** is necessary for the allergic person because it builds the nervous system which is under great stress during allergic reactions. **Yeast, an allergen implicated in many allergy responses, is the prime source of many B-complex for-**

mulas. Buy "rice based" B-complex formulas for allergic persons. Finally, **N-Dimethylglycine or DMG,** commonly misnamed B_{15}, is excellent for increasing the amount of oxygen available to cells (helps a person breathe and also increases energy. **Suggested dosages for the average adult allergy person per day:**

  Vitamin C Ascorbate - 2,000-5,000 mg.
  Panthothenic Acid - 500 mg./3 times per day
  DMG - 2-4 tablets as needed to breath
  B-Complex - 2 tablets twice a day (high potency rice based).
  Calcium - (orotate, gluconate, no lactate) - 1,000 mg at
      bedtime
  Magnesium (orotate) - 500 mg. at breakfast
  Vitamin E - 100 I.U. to 200 I.U. (d-alpha tocopherols).

After the allergic symptoms are under control, reduce the adrenal support supplements to half, but continue the limited use of milk products, wheat and oranges.

Supplementation for allergic children:

  Vitamin C Ascorbate - 1,000-3,000 mg.
  Panthothenic Acid - 250 mg./3 times per day
  DMG - 2 tablets a day
  B-complex - 2 tablets a day (high potency rice based)
  Calcium - 500 mg. at bedtime
  Magnesium Orotate - 250 mg. at breakfast
  Vitamin E - 100 I.U. with meals

Although supplements can aid the body in building immunity to allergens, **the dietary changes recommended in this book are essential so that these supplements will be absorbed properly** (see Chapter Five).

CHAPTER 10

STRESS: HOW TO COPE

"ROW, ROW, ROW YOUR BOAT, GENTLY DOWN THE STREAM . . ."

Properly defined, **stress is an adaptive response in which the body prepares or adjusts to a threatening situation.**

Many people think that stress is the actual person, place, circumstance or thing that upsets them. Actually factors such as getting caught in a traffic jam, working non-stop at a feverish pace, eating the wrong foods or losing a job are **stressors,** not stress. Even emotions such as rage, hate, anger, nervous tension or frustration are stressors, not stress.

All of the above **stressors** threaten your body as a whole, forcing it to make certain chemical and physiological changes in order to resist or adapt to the stressor presented.

Stress has subtle effects on the endocrine glands (hormones), nervous system, and immunological system. When a stressor triggers the stress mechanism, the body activates all of its defenses into an organized response. Although the body often does not know what triggered the response, it nevertheless resists. The pituitary, hypothalamus (primitive portion of the brain involved in gut-level responses), and adrenal glands begin to function at an increased rate. **The adrenals, because they work so closely with the nervous system, are more affected than any other gland during a stressful situation.** These glands sit on top of the kidneys and have been known to enlarge in order to produce additional hormones or flatten like pancakes during complete exhaustion. **When the adrenals exhaust, the body has no defense against the stressors of daily living.**

During stress, hormone production increases, particularly adrenal cortical output. Other glands and organs such as the thyroid, liver and heart begin to overwork. Additionally, output of red and white blood cells increase in order to fight infection, blood sugar rises offering more energy to cells and blood pressure increases as the heart tries to compensate by moving more blood, oxygen and nutrients into muscles and tissues. **Furthermore, a retention of water often results as salt is collected in the tissues and the body actually increases fat storage as toxins are moved to the outer tissues.**

Nutritional needs of the body skyrocket during stress. Resistance falls in direct proportion to the depletion of Vitamin C reserves, which are greatly taxed during stressful periods. Vitamin C is the first vitamin to come under stress in any tissue. During stress, Vitamin E, pantothenic acid, Vitamin A and all the B-vitamins are used up in massive amounts. The body withdraws minerals from its bones, teeth, hair, organs and other tissues to meet the demands of defense. The body breaks down protein from itself to create more hormones and antibodies. Calcium, magnesium, phosphorous and potassium demands are also increased under stress. As hydrochloric acid production decreases under stress, protein metabolism becomes impaired. Respiratory infections, stomach distress and constipation increase as resistance decreases. Allergies develop as resistance falls.

As the body becomes deficient in essential nutrients, its ability to resist the stressors diminishes. If a stress is prolonged for weeks, months or years, the body is unable to convert cholesterol into needed hormones. Such continued stress results in complete exhaustion and total collapse. **"Nervous breakdowns", heart attacks, cancers, strokes, liver damage or kidney damage are examples of complete exhaustion caused by constant stress.**

Unfortunately, many people realize the need for an improved lifestyle only after a heart attack, arthritic attack or nervous breakdown. **The accumulating affects of "wear and tear" due to stress over a sufficient time period (which varies with each individual) may lead to the two major degenerative diseases — cancer and/or heart disease.**

In days past, stressors were easily recognized and resolutions were possible. If I came upon a tiger in the woods, my response system would trigger sufficient adrenaline and energy enabling me to either fight the tiger or swiftly retreat.

After the stress passed, my body's response mechanisms would return to normal. However, in today's hectic environment, many stressors are not identifiable or resolvable. If someone pulls out in front of my car during rush hour traffic and I swerve to avoid a possible accident, my adrenals are quickly activated. I cannot even "chew" the driver out, and consequently, continue to harbor anger and resentment for the rest of the day. **Many people are "on the defensive," prepared to protect themselves against unknown assailants and ready to fight (verbally or physically) at the drop of a hat.** The body is not designed to be on **"Red Alert"** all the time and will eventually exhaust under such strain. **The unresolvable stress overload is the cause of many illnesses and deaths in the United States.**

We cannot change many of the modern stressors we face daily, but we can change our responses to them. Eating patterns can be modified in order to help a person cope with the stress of modern day living. The **"Optimum Diet for Optimum Health,"** along with an exercise program and supplements, will provide such a person with the "bank account" so important in the twentieth century. **A body in optimum health is prepared for stress and able to respond with the needed energy to cope with life.**

Although a nutrition program is a vital compontent of protection against the depletion that stress causes, combining other aspects to raise resistance can produce a much greater effect. **The following are suggestions for increasing resistance in your body by developing strategies for coping with stress.**

1. **An Exercise Program** - helps both psychologically and physiologically "burn off' or release stressful situations that occur on a daily basis (see Chapter 11).

2. **Quiet Time** - Everyone needs to have a few minutes alone where the noise and demands of others are put aside. Solitude is at a premium in today's crowded world. Take a quiet walk in the park or retreat into a private room where only the sound of silence can be heard. A few minutes of quiet time will recharge the frayed nerves of a tension-filled day.

3. **Commune with your Creator** - I am a firm believer in the need for human beings to spend time in religious and spiritual pursuits. Reading religious books such as the Bible, praying or meditating are all effective means to quiet the restless mind and heal the feelings of separation and aliena- tion so common in today's fragmented existence. Take time to make a connection with the source of your life and be thankful for all your Creator has given you.

4. **Develop a Positive Attitude** - "If life hands you a lemon, learn to make lemonaid." Have you ever noticed how your life changes? People, places and events rarely remain the same. When something in your life causes anger or pain, say to yourself, **"This too shall pass,"** for it most certainly will. Hold fast, hold fast, the night will not last.

5. **Learn to Love** - Love is the greatest nutrient and most powerful healer you will ever experience. Give your time, wholeheartedly, to your family, your friends and those less fortunate than yourself. Notice how your problems are less overwhelming or hopeless when you are helping others. Love fills a person with a wonderful feeling that is priceless. **Whenever possible give someone a hug.** The latest research suggests we need twelve hugs a day to maintain good health. A hug can be given anytime, anyplace and to anyone. If hugs cost ten thousand dollars, more people would probably want one; but alas, they are free. Remember, hugs are non- fattening, 100% organic and natural, cure depression, reduce stress, have no unpleasant side effects and improve the body's immune system. **The doctor of the future will tell you to "give 2 hugs and call me in the morning." If there are no humans around to hug, get an animal.** Studies confirm in- teraction with pets like dogs or cats prolong the life and hap- piness of people confined to nursing homes. Other studies show that prisoners allowed to keep small pets such as cag- ed birds or hamsters are much less likely to attack fellow in- mates or commit suicide. A pet acts as a catalyst for giving and receiving affection. Patients in and out of hospitals recover more quickly from illnesses and diseases when they interact with pets. **Much of the healing power of pets seems**

to be the pet's ability to make a person laugh while offering dependable, unconditional love and companionship.

6. **Learn to Play** - Our world is so serious. The starving millions, the atomic bomb, the devastating effects of drugs and the high inflation make play seem a privilege of children only. Play means participating in something non-rational or even silly; play is just good old-fashioned, clean fun. Play is a time when a person can forget about the horrors of war and the decline of civilization, and enjoy the simple, uninhibited pleasures of life without the need for alcohol or drugs. In order to begin to play, think of something that you've always wanted to do (shouldn't cost over $10.00), and do it. Attend a funny movie that will make you laugh until your sides ache, or invite your friends over for a friendly game of volleyball. **The doctor of the future will prescribe one hour a day of play to reduce stress and improve health.**

7. **Develop a Close Friend** - Do you have a friend that you can share anything with. A friend is someone who doesn't judge you, and hears every word you want to say. A friend is a person you can tell all your "deep, dark secrets" to, share your hopes and dreams with and laugh and cry with. Even if you don't see them for weeks or years you never lose the closeness. If you have a real friend, be truly thankful, for they help you relieve the stresses of your life.

CONCLUSION

A diet of optimum foods, vitamin supplementation, and a lifestyle consisting of exercise, quiet time, positive attitude, spiritual commitment, close friends and love will help you respond more positively to stress.

Permit the stresses of your life to be your teachers. A heart attack may seem like a tragedy, and yet, this experience may be the crisis you need to take a healthier direction in your life. The psoriasis I experienced at an early age in my life motivated me to become a Nutrition Consultant and to share my findings with you in this book.

CHAPTER 11

EXERCISE: USE IT OR LOSE IT

"YOUR BODY IS THE ONE MACHINE THAT WORKS BETTER THE MORE IT IS USED."

"If you permit your automobile to stand idle for a few years, the engine and body begin to corrode and rust. **Remember that too much rest brings rusts.** Action is a law of health. Every organ in the body must work in order to maintain strength and vitality, while stagnation will cause decay and death.

The marriage of exercise and diet is absolutely essential if the Lazy Person wishes to experience optimum health and energy. **Exercise improves blood circulation; and the blood is the carrier of all the nutrients you eat.** As nutritious food and supplements are digested, vitamins, minerals, proteins, carbohydrates and fat are absorbed through the walls of the small intestine and directed into the bloodstream. If circulation is good, the nutrients will be transported via the blood to every organ, gland and cell.

The bottom line of the Nutrition Game is to feed the cells of your body. Your body contains trillions of cells making up every organ, gland and tissue. Cells digest food and eliminate waste, just like you do. They are born, reproduce and die, and if they receive the nutrients they need to perform their appointed tasks, your whole body feels alive and well. **Exercise is crucial to the proper nutrition of your cells.**

Exercise improves your metabolism. Recently exercise such as jogging, walking, swimming, cycling and aerobic dance have become very popular. With their increased popularity, new research concerning exercise physiology has been developed. Current studies indicate that a person who exercises regularly can increase his/her metabolism (the rate at which cells use energy or calories) up to 30%!

A regular exercise program improves your tone, circulation, organ functions, digestion, absorbtion and elimination. **Exer-

cise is the best digestive aid you can take. Instead of using digestive enzyme supplements to improve food assimilation, take a brisk walk! There is no supplement that can replace all the benefits of regular, aerobic exercise. And most importantly, you will enforce the important nutritional law, **"You are what you assimilate."**

Modern civilization, with all its conveniences, has brought with it less and less activity. Automobiles, buses, escalators, elevators, washing machines, television, office work and countless hours of sitting has transformed a once beautiful, graceful, erect and slender physical specimen into what many have become today. Rounded shoulders, poor muscle tone, pale faces, "pot bellies," stiff and inflexible joints, aching feet and obesity are a few consequences of the inactivity of modern living. **Each muscle joint was meant for use,** and if you do not find time to exercise, you become sluggish and fatigued.

The greatest pick-me-up is not a cup of coffee or a candy bar, but exercise. Exercise makes you feel good all over and relieves tension, too! Our lives are filled with stress, and exercise is the key ingredient to daily release. Exercise is also one of the greatest remedies for depression and worry. Additionally, your energy level is boosted for two hours after exercising, making it the best prescription for fatigue!

BENEFITS OF EXERCISE

1. Speeds up circulation, keeps blood cruising through the body
2. Improves food digestion and speeds up a sluggish metabolism
3. Improves strength and function of all internal organs/glands
4. Removes lactic acid and other poisons from the body by improving elimination of the skin, lungs and bowels
5. Eliminates constipation
6. Builds coordination, balance and improves reflexes
7. Helps maintain a tranquil mind
8. Keeps muscles fit, trim and flexible
9. Reduces risks of developing heart disease, obesity, arteriosclerosis and high blood pressure

10. Brings more oxygen into every cell of the body
11. Improves sleep patterns
12. Gives the opportunity to spend quality time with yourself every day
13. Creates the opportunity to be outside
14. Enables you to meet new friends
15. Reduces the tendency to overeat
16. Releases the stresses of the day
17. Increases energy
18. It is a positive means of escape

By developing the daily habit of exercise, you will feel and look better. Your body is poorly built for sitting and not much better for standing, but for walking, running and swimming, it is superb.

The most important thing to remember in the beginning of an exercise program is that it is as essential to your health as eating, breathing, sleeping or loving. **Since exercise must be done throughout your entire life choose a program you enjoy.** We are developing a lifestyle to improve and promote optimum health in the **Lazy Person's Guide,** and enjoyment is a key to maintaining that lifestyle.

WHAT KIND OF EXERCISE?

Include an aerobic exercise. An aerobic exercise is steady and nonstop movement for a duration of at least 12 minutes (30 minutes is recommended). An intensity of 50% to 80% of maximum heart rate constitutes proper conditioning. The way to compute maximum heart rate is to subtract your age from 220.

220 - Your Age = Maximum Heart Rate

Multiply .80 x Maximum Heart Rate and you have the rate fitness experts recommend for achieving an aerobic peak. Sustaining this rate for twelve minutes will insure an increased oxygen and blood flow.

Include stretching and flexibility exercises as part of your daily or weekly program. The more flexible and strong your body, the less likely you are to be prone to "pain and injury." A series of stretching exercises will keep your muscles well toned.

Here are a few aerobic exercises presented for your consideration:

WALKING

Walking is probably the most natural and oldest form of exercise. Walking can be started at any age and maintained throughout your life. Because it is less strenuous than other forms of exercise, the chance of injury is less. While walking, almost all of your muscles are utilized, your abdominal muscles are tightened and strengthened and you can experience permanent weight loss. 3,500 calories must be burnt to lose one pound. A one hour walk every other day at a moderate pace (three miles an hour) will burn 300 to 360 calories. In other words, you can burn up a pound and a half a month, or 18 pounds a year, providing there is no food intake change. If you wish to lose weight faster, walk an hour a day everyday and burn up three pounds a month of 36 pounds a year.

REBOUNDER

Utilization of the small, round trampoline designed for home or office use is an excellent way to exercise indoors. Jumping and jogging on a rebounder will stimulate circulation, heart rate, elimination and enhance fat burning for weight loss and weight control. And you can listen to music or watch your favorite television program while you jump. Half an hour, twice a day, is ideal to maintain you energy and health (see Video List).

JOGGING

The word "jog" literally means "to jar." Subjecting your body to a daily regime of pounding on asphalt or cement, bruising kidneys, liver, reproductive organs, knees, lower back and ankles does not sound like the Lazy Person's way to maintain good health.

Instead, find a beautiful park, country road or golf course where you can run on grass or dirt. This practice reduces the stress on the muscular/skeletal system, as well as the kidneys. Stretch 10 minutes before your run and 20 minutes afterwards to reduce sprains and other injuries caused by shortening muscles. Buy the proper shoes too!

SWIMMING

Lap swimming is an excellent aerobic endurance workout. However, do not expect to lose much weight as the body will retain fat in order to maintain body heat in the water. Swimmers have a larger percentage of body fat than any other aerobic exerciser. If possible, avoid chlorinated pools.

CYCLING

Cycling can be a fine aerobic exercise if done on a lap basis like swimming. Unfortunately, many people "coast" a significant amount of the time while riding, resulting in little actual exercise. For maximum results, find a bike path or park where you can build up speed for a continuous amount of time.

JUMPING ROPE

This form of exercise, like trampoline, is an excellent winter, indoor sport. Ten minutes of jumping rope is equivalent to 30 minutes of jogging, and helps maintain good circulation and weight loss. If possible, jump on a thick rug to eliminate muscular/skeletal system jarring.

Some studies indicate that aerobic exercise decreases appetite by regulating your appestat, the brain center that controls appetite. These studies show that bloodflow is redirected away from the digestive tract, stimulating the muscular use of blood fats instead of blood sugars. Unfortunately, the importance of somatopsychic physiology and medicine is not yet adequately appreciated. A five mile walk does more for an unhappy, but otherwise healthy person, than all the tranquilizers possible. And no side effects other than good health! Stress can be counteracted and even prevented by regular, vigorous exercise. In other words, **exercise is Nature's antidote for nervous conditions.**

According to Covert Bailey, author of <u>Fit Or Fat</u>:

1. Fitness is **lost** if you exercise **two days** or less a week
2. Fitness is **maintained** if you exercise **four days** a week
3. Fitness is **improved** if you exercise **six days** a week

IMPORTANT

People with hypoglycemic symptoms should exercise moderately (less strenuously, but longer duration) so the liver will convert glycogen into glucose and raise the blood sugar level rather then short, strenuous exercise which reduces the sugar in the blood.

CONCLUSION

Recent studies found that people who exercise regularly generally felt better than those who exercised less, unless they ate lots of sweets, fast food and coffee. The junk food junkies, regardless of how much they exercise, reported greater levels of fatigue and problems with memory and sleep. The moral of this study: exercise is not a cure-all. You must eat right too, if you want to feel really good. If you marry the Optimum Diet For Optimum Health with a regular exercise program you will experience greater energy and vitality.

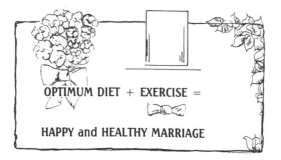

OPTIMUM DIET + EXERCISE =

HAPPY and HEALTHY MARRIAGE

The Lazy Person's Guide recommends exercising **at least 30 minutes daily, six days weekly for best results.** Begin your exercise program **today,** but remember to **start moderately** and increase intensity and duration as you get in better shape. Your are in no hurry, but **exercise as if your life depends on it, because it does!**

CAUTION: SEE YOUR PHYSICIAN BEFORE BEGINNING ANY EXERCISE PROGRAM.

CHAPTER 12

YOUR QUESTIONS ANSWERED BY GORDON TESSLER PH.D.

Q. I am reading magazine articles claiming the value of pasta. Is this an acceptable alternative to eating grains?

A. Alas, no. Although pasta is made from whole grains (such as wheat), and vegetables (such as spinach), pasta is a processed food! Pasta is not a good fiber food like **whole** grains are and acts more like glue constipating your intestines. Pasta can be eaten once a month as a "binging food", but there is no substitute for complex carbohydrates. Grains provide both energy and **a moving experience.** Unless you run several miles a day to burn up the calories and keep the bowels going, watch out for pasta!

Q. Can I use vinegar?

A. If your system is not over-acid, vinegar may be included in your diet. Use only apple cider vinegar. White vinegar should be avoided as its harshness is said to kill red blood cells (iron and oxygen carrying cells) in your body.

Q. Describe the symptoms of PMS (Pre-Menstrual Syndrome) and are there any natural remedies for it?

A. There are physical symptoms such as severe cramping, headaches, nausea, bloating, water retention, sweet cravings and fatigue. The more serious implications of PMS are psychological and emotional. Depression, crying spells, anger, resentment, hostility and impatience, to name a few. During a menstrual cycle, a woman can loose 40 times more calcium and magnesium than in any other time of the month. B-complex and particularly B_6 known for its diuretic properties, brain stimulation, and female hormonal properties are also lost. PMS is a classic example of certain essential nutrient deficiencies creating symptomatic problems. A few drugless clinics in the United States are using B-complex, B_6, calcium and magnesium as well as a complex carbohydrate diet to correct this condition.

The use of refined sugar not only depletes the B-complex calcium and magnesium of a womans body, but also increases the cravings for sugar, particularly during the menstrual cycle. Eliminating refined sugar and adding the above mentioned nutrients is a safe and effective means of ending PMS.

Q. I read so much about kelp in all the health magazines. Is it as good as people say? Is there any danger in taking it?

A. Kelp is a seaweed very rich in natural iodine. Iodine is essential to the function of the thyroid gland. It is also a rich source of such essential minerals as calcium, magnesium, sodium and potassium, One of the proported properties of kelp is its ability to remove X-rays or radiation from our bodies. Because of the ability that kelp has of attracting radiation, pacific kelp is high in radioactive material. There is now some question about kelp grown in Japan. (You remember a bomb was dropped there not too long ago.) My suggestion is to buy Norwegian Kelp to insure there is no radioactive danger. Seaweed grown in the far northern part of our hemisphere is the best.

Women should consider another seaweed called dulse because of its richer concentration of potassium.

Q. Is honey better for you than sugar?

A. No, not really. Honey is a simple invert sugar with traces of B vitamins and vitamin C. Invert sugar is usually a combination of glucose and fructose. White sugar is sucrose but becomes invert sugar when our bodies break it down. Honey, being a simple sugar, can also contribute to hypoglycemic symptoms. Honey tastes twice as sweet as regular table sugar. Because of its stickiness, honey clings to the teeth and unless removed promptly with brushing, will promote tooth decay faster than sugar does. A better sugar substitute is apple juice concentrate or barley malt syrup.

Q. Is it natural as we get older to lose our memory?

A. As a matter of fact, I had a client last week tell me that they were losing their memory and could I help them? I in turn asked, "When did this conditon begin?" And the client replied, "When did what condition begin?"

There are a few vitamins and minerals which are essential to memory and are easily lost in processing, over-cooking and eating junk food. Potassium, which is essential to sending electrical impulses during the thought process, is easily depleted in the American diet by the use of alcohol, salt and coffee. Magnesium is essential to the nerve impulses and muscles and is robbed from the body by the use of sugar, coffee and alcohol. B_6, another brain vitamin, can be robbed from our bodies by the use of pop, diet or otherwise (containing phosphoric acid, the thief of B_6) as well as sugar, coffee and alcohol. The use of table salt also constricts and hardens the arteries making blood and oxygen flow to the brain very difficult. Obviously the longer you've lived, the more salt you've consumed and the worse the problem can become. The need for daily aerobic exercise to clean out the arteries and improve circulation is a positive addiction that we Americans are just beginning to understand. A combination of the above nutritional deficiencies and lack of exercise are most of the cause of loss of memory. The lack of adequate zinc in the diet can cause memory problems, as well as aluminum toxicity.

Q. I've been reading about how healthy fasting is and I've done a few short fasts. I became not only very hungry, but sick to my stomach and very, very tired. What am I doing wrong.

A. Fasting has been used since Biblical times for spiritual and therapeutic purposes. Today, however, fasting is used mostly for maintaining weight control. One day we eat junk food, the second day we fast, and the third day we turn over a new leaf and eat natural food. Eratic and extreme eating habits, cause more harm than good. Fasting can be very beneficial if done with supervision and planning. During a fast, blood sugar decreases and if a person suffers from hypoglycemia or low blood sugar, they may experience the symptoms you have just mentioned. **Don't fast if you suspect you have low blood sugar.** Instead learn to eat complex carbohydrates (grains) and small frequent meals. Eating 3-6 raw almonds every hour and a half will help control your blood sugar. The word fasting means resting, so if you feel ready to do a fast, take a vacation from your daily stressful life.

Q. Medical reports indicate that the sun is very harmful and that you should avoid it and I've also heard that the sun is a healing agent, and fights infection. Can you help me? I'm confused.

A. Sunlight has been used throughout history as a means to control or help fight infections. The white blood cell and lymphocyte counts in the blood, both infection fighters, increase after 1/2 hour of sunbathing. Niels Finsen in the early 1900's found that test tubes full of a destructive bacteria multiplied while setting in dark areas of his lab, while those test tubes placed in the window of his lab, exposed to the sun, destroyed the bacteria. He re-discovered an ancient truth - **the sun is a healer.** A series of successful remissions of patients with skin tuberculosis followed. Exposure to the sun for specific periods of time caused these patients to become well. A Nobel Prize followed these findings. But remember only mad dogs go out in the noonday sun. The burning rays which can contribute to skin cancer are most powerful from 10 a.m. to 3 p.m. My suggestion would be to sunbathe between the hours of 7 and 9 a.m. and after 4 p.m. These are the safest and most beneficial hours to reap the healing powers of the sun.

Arthritics find relief for their painful joints by sunbathing regularly. Sunlight also reduces the cholesterol levels in the blood. Cholesterol readings were reduced by more than 30 points with patients exposed for as little as 30 minutes in the sun. Few people are aware that Vitamin D is manufactured on the skin by exposure to the sun rays. Vitamin D helps the absorption and utilization of calcium in our bodies. Through exposure to the suns rays, cholesterol and other fats are brought out of the blood to the surface of the skin where these oils produce Vitamin D.

Suggestion - Do not shower for at least 30 minutes after exposure to the sun, for you will wash away these important oils before your body can absorb the Vitamin D.

Q.   I have been on every kind of weight loss diet that's in existence and have lost more than 1,000 lbs. in my lifetime. Unfortunately, I have also gained more than a 1,000 lbs. in my lifetime. Is there an alternative?

A.   An overweight person must **develop a lifestyle including exercise and nutrition** to take weight off safely and permanently. Unfortunately, lifestyle changes take time, but so did putting on the weight. A healthy weight loss for a person that is 20-30 lbs. overweight should be no more than 8 lbs. a month. Eat 8-10 small meals a day using raw unsalted almonds as a between meal snack. Eliminate all refined carbohydrates including sugar, breads, spaghetti, lasagna, etc. and replace these empty starches with complex carbohydrates such as oats, brown rice, millet, and barley. This will insure that a person gets the sugar the body needs without going **"starch-craving mad."** Also eliminate salt from your diet. This will insure that you won't retain excess water. Eliminate milk and hard cheese, and replace with a plain, unsweetened yogurt. A high-fiber, complex carbohydrate diet, will improve the elimination of the bowels and help flatten out the stomach.

Metabolic imbalances of the pancreas and thyroid, as well as hormonal imbalances can also contribute to a poor metabolism (see your nutritionist for metabolic evaluation). Exercise, particularly aerobic activity for 30 minutes, 6 days a week will help speed up a sluggish metabolism. The above considerations are the only sure way to healthy and balanced weight control.

Q.   Is margarine really better for you than butter?

A.   Vegetable oil at room temperature is a liquid, so the question is why is margarine solid at room temperature? A process called hydrogenation is a chemical process where hydrogenated molecules are forced into the molecular structure of the vegetable margarine. A temperature of 300 degrees is required. The use of margarine, although it has no cholesterol, is still a dangerous alternative since these partially hydrogenated vegetable oils cannot be effectively broken down by the human body. This fat accumulates in the arteries and over works the liver and gall bladder. Small amounts of **unsalted butter** in our diet is a much more natural and healthy practice. (1 to 2 pats a day).

Q. I have had an iron deficiency all my life. What should I do?

A. Iron is an essential component of hemoglobin and transporter of oxygen. Calcium and vitamin C are necessary for the metabolism of iron in the human body. Such deficiency symptoms as weakness, skin pallor, anemia, fatigue, menstrual irregularity, loss of strength, constipation, brittle nails, dizziness, and respiration problems can result from a lack of iron. Even when serum blood levels of iron are adequate, the cellular absorption may be low due to insufficient vitamin C and calcium intake in the diet. **Floradix,** a natural liquid iron, is a good supplement, as well as calcium **ascorbate** for increased vitamin C utilization.

Q. Is too much exercise as dangerous as too little?

A. As a matter of fact, yes. Recent studies at several universities indicate that over-exercise can lower hormone levels in men and women. Particularly in the case of women, jogging even as little as 2 miles, 5 times a week can cause less estrogen to be produce. This condition can lead to P.M.S. (premenstrual syndrome) as well as infrequent menstruation. Some lady runners say that their periods stop for months or even years when strenuous activity is maintained. Mens' levels of testosterone are reduced when strenuous activity is maintained resulting in diminished sex drive. **Be moderate in all things, even good ones.**

Q. Is coffee drinking related to kidney stones? My husband has had 3 stones in the past 2 years and drinks a lot of coffee.

A. Coffee contains oxalic acid, which can be very damaging to the kidneys and stomach. Calcium and magnesium, buffers of heavy acids in the body, attempt to neutralize this oxalic acid. If the body is forced to continually neutralize this acid, stones may form. Kidney stones consist of calcium oxide (calcium-oxalic acid) and magnesium oxide (magnesium-oxalic acid). Since commercial "de cafs" are rich in oxalic acid and are decaffinated with a carcinogenic chemical, they are not good alternatives.

Q. Ever since my divorce 7 years ago, when I gained thirty pounds, I can't seem to lose weight. I tried many high protein diets and although I do lose some weight, I always gain it back. What can I do?

A. Your frustration is shared by many women in the United States. Food has become a dear friend during stressful times or crisis situations. Unless we deal with feelings which cause us to over-eat, we will never obtain a permanent weight loss. For instance, during a stressful divorce (and what divorce is not?) a person may feel anger, emptiness, fear, loneliness, and/or depression. One way to deal with these painful feelings is to eat "reward" type foods. Suppose during this period a person ate a lot of chocolate and gained thirty pounds. After the divorce, perhaps a year later, this person wants to lose that thirty pounds. As the pounds come off, the feelings of anger, etc. resurface. Through therapy and counseling you can deal with these emotions, instead of stuffing them down with food. **A successful and permanent weight loss includes an honest resolution of these inner hungers.**

Q. If I am a "good" person with my diet most of the time, do I lose ground by binging over the Holidays?

A. Aboslutely not! It is not what a person does occasionally that determines health or disease, but what a person does **most** of the time. Enjoy your Holidays, **and learn** to make healthier "goodies".

Q.   I read a lot about the importance of zinc in the diet. Is its importance overestimated?

A.   Zinc is an essential nutrient in the human body. Studies have shown zinc and B_6 supplementation can regulate menstrual cycles, as well as restore normal sexual function in impotent young males who are zinc deficient. Zinc supplementation in zinc deficient patients promotes wound healing when given both pre and post-operatively. Joint pain and circulation may be helped by zinc supplementation. Zinc may aid in healing stretch marks on hips, thighs, abdomen, breasts and shoulder girdles. Food processing and over-cooking, as well as consumption of fast foods, all contribute to zinc deficiencies. Smoking and alcohol are very damaging to zinc levels. Today our soil lacks zinc because it is water soluable and excessive rainfall can leach zinc from our soil.

Foods like pumpkin seeds, sunflower seeds and nuts contain good sources of zinc provided they are not roasted and/or salted. (If you have white spots on your fingernails, this could indicate zinc deficiency.)

Q.   Dr. Airola and other authorities advocate Brewer's Yeast for B-complex. How much should I take?

A.   None. Recent studies indicate yeast of all kinds including the sacred panacea-Brewer's Yeast, is an allergy food. After all, yeast is a mold! Brewer's Yeast is 50% protein which renders it very difficult to digest. A well known nutritionist claimed that if you experienced gas while taking Brewer's Yeast, you needed it! If you experience gas and flatulence from yeast, you can't digest it. Use Rice Polish instead to supplement your B-complex needs.

Q.   With all the controversy over hair analysis, is the test really valid.

A.   Absolutely. One of the primary objections to hair analysis is that the results aren't consistent. A few years ago some experiments were done where a sample of hair was sent to 5 hair laboratories and the results turned out to be not only different, but contradictory. One lab reported normal calcium, another lab reported low calcium and still another reported high calcium.

The problems with these laboratories reporting different results were fourfold:

1. Various state-of-the-art machinery to perform tests.
2. Solvents used to prepare hair for analysis were different.
3. Quality control varied.
4. Procedures of cutting hair for samples varied.

A board has been set up to regulate and **standardize** the many hair labs across the country and separate the legitimate ones from the "flaky" ones. The cost of hair analysis is an indication of a laboratory's hair-analysis technology. A photo-spectrometer, the best procedure for accessing minerals is a costly, but precise means of receiving reliable and compatible data from different laboratories. The industry is regulating itself very reputably, although I still only recommend a few hair-mineral labs in the United States.

Q. I am a working mother with a two-year-old daughter. I am almost always busy. But in addition to what I accomplish now, I am planning on attending college. I would be interested in learning which foods will help me concentrate on my studies and enable me to stay awake in the evenings when I will have to study late after my daughter is in bed. Thank you in advance for your advice.

A. First, it is vitally important that a person who wishes good, clear brain power and concentration not use concentrated or refined sugars. These sugars would include white and brown sugar, honey, molasses, maple syrup and corn syrup. Concentrated sugar requires a **high insulin response** which **lowers** blood sugar abruptly; leaving a person tired, confused, depressed and forgetful. Since our brains need an abundance of glucose (sugar) to function optimally, the sugars best suited for brain efficiency are complex carbohydrates, i.e. grains, legumes, seeds and nuts. Grains such as oats, brown rice, millet, buckwheat, rye and barley, release glucose over an extended period (3-6 hours), stabilizing the blood sugar for a corresponding length of time. Grains are superior sources of thiamin B_1, riboflavin B_2, niacin B_3, pantothenic acid B_5, pyridoxine B_6, and protein, all crucial to proper brain-nervous system function. Also grains are rich in all minerals needed for optimum brain function.

Eating grains for breakfast as well as lunch or dinner plus snacking on raw, unsalted almonds between meals will insure enough brain energy to study late into the evening.

Q. I am overweight and I would like to fast to lose some unwanted pounds. How long should I fast? Should I do a water fast? Should I take my supplements during my fast?

A. Part of developing a philosophy of living in harmony with the laws of nature, as practiced by healthy cultures, is to learn the importance of correct fasting.

In a country of plenty, where most living is done in excess, an occassional abstinence from eating gives the entire digestive system a well-deserved vacation. Animals, in their natural habitat, have periods of fasting due to changes of season or sickness. In Europe, many resorts and sanitariums conduct fasting regimes to correct illness and disease. Fasting is also very beneficial, especially in the spring, to detoxify and cleanse winter gluttony.

Fasting on fruit and vegetable juices rather than water will help maintain steady blood sugar levels. If a person is intending a 3-day fast or longer, a few days of fruit and vegetables only, will prepare your body for the fast to come.

Also breaking a fast is very crucial. For every three days you fast, one day of eating light foods is necessary after the fast. Foods like meat, dairy and nuts should be avoided during the light eating days.

During a fast, the body begins to detoxify drugs, uric acid, environmental poisons and mucus out of every cell, tissue and organ. An **enema** everyday is absolutely vital to this cleansing process otherwise a fast can do much harm due to the accumulation of toxins in the liver, kidneys and bowel. Juices and teas should add up to one **gallon** of liquid per day during the fast to assist the body, especially the kidneys in the elimination process. Since vitamins are best absorbed with food, **do not take vitamins during fasting periods.**

Fasting is a wonderful and healthful practice, which leaves a person feeling great. Fast means rest, so don't try to keep up normal working hours. Relax and enjoy. Read Dr. Airola's, How To Stay Slim, Healthy And Young Through Juice Fasting, before beginning any fast.

CHAPTER 13

DEAR DR. TESSLER - THANK YOU.....

"There are three kinds of people:
1. The people who **make** things happen.
2. The people who **watch** things happen.
3. The people who **wonder** what happened."

Dear Dr. Tessler,

It was a "red letter" day for me when I tuned into an early morning talk show and heard you speak. At the time I was suffering from an extreme case of bronchial asthma and being treated with Prednisone, Tebutaline, and Theodore, to mention a few. I had been cautioned about the side-effects these medications had, and they really weren't helping me all that much. Many times I had to be rushed to the hospital when the attacks would be so acute I feared for my life. Being sick became a way of life for me. I could barely walk up a few steps without gasping for breath — to say nothing of trying to walk from my car to the office in cold weather. When I could lie down to sleep, I usually awakened wheezing and gasping for breath; I'd finish out the night by hanging over a chair. Naturally, I was in bad shape to face another day of business when this happened — and it happened all too frequently.

Listening to you speak that morning, I realized that you were talking about people who were in my category, and it gave me enough hope to call and make an appointment to see you. The first thing I discovered was that my eating habits were all wrong. Although I ate a balanced diet at mealtime, I also ate a lot of "junk" food in between — and being in business, I often skipped by regular meals. My "balanced diet" also proved to contain many things that were harmful to me — as I later learned under your guidance. You advised me to take many vitamins and minerals, along with a sensible mode of eating. Fish and chicken replaced steaks and chops, etc. that I thought were so good for me. You educated me in the proper diet for my particular problem, and in fact, even had your staff conduct food preparation sessions which were very helpful. After having lived three-fourths of my life with bad eating habits, I thought the transition would be difficult. But when I had a choice of breathing or not — it wasn't difficult at all.

There are so many interesting ways to prepare fish and chicken — using herbs instead of salt and pepper — that I'm never really bored with my menus. It doesn't bother me at all to see others enjoying the desserts that I once ate with gusto, because I know that the ingredients could be poison to my body. Before I revised my eating habits, I was so depressed with having to live the way I felt — and having to fight to breath — that I thought death would be a welcome alternative. With my present regime, and being able to exercise again, I now feel that life is worth living. I haven't had any medication for over two-and-one-half years (when I first started coming to you), and feel better than I have in ages. I can't say enough about how important good eating habits, vitamins and minerals have been to my well being, and I will never forget my good fortune in tuning in to that talk show nearly three years ago. I'll always be grateful to you for giving me a new lease on life — and showing me how to maintain it.

Dear Dr. Tessler,

Up until 3 1/2 years ago, I've been fighting and ignoring a degenerating disease called Muscular Dystrophy, with no knowledge of the amazing abilities that our bodies have to heal itself with the proper nutrition, exercise and attitude.

All my life I've been slowly destroying my body by flooding it with bad foods, drugs and alcohol.

To make a long story short, my arms and shoulders became very weak through my junior high years and my hips and thighs became weaker during my high school years. By the time I was 23 years old, I was walking with my hands in my back pockets to support my hips.

Moving to Colorado with my sister June was very interesting. Dr. Gordon put me in a body cast so I could walk and put me in a therapy program. After nine months of free weights, I became so much stronger that everyone was impressed. I reached a point and stayed there not getting better or worse, but I was encouraged to go on.

Two years later, my sister June died of cancer and I was living by myself, still drinking and doing drugs. I met this nutritionist who told me I could run again if I followed a certain program.

Within 2 months I quit drinking, drugs and all processed foods, along with what most people eat daily. It wasn't so easy as 1-2-3, but I don't have time or space to go into detail. Regardless, after 2 1/2 years I turned into another person in body and soul. This time everyone was astounded at the change. I was walking, swimming and doing nautilus much better. My muscles were getting stronger!

Then I met you. After some tests, we found my body was depleted in certain minerals. So by putting together certain massive doses of minerals and vitamins my body started to absorb these nutrients within weeks (I'm not exaggerating at all). I was walking 3 times more and with much more coordination! The next year I started to work out 2 1/2 hours a day instead of one!

It's a slow process, but I figure my alternatives are not very select. I used to run and jump all the time and I plan on doing it again. Just think — if all this can help a body in my condition, think what good nutrition could do for the average Joe!

Dear Dr. Tessler,

I want to write a few lines to tell you how much I have benefited from your nutrition program.

I have been on the program now for about eight months, and I feel that it has helped me greatly. For years I have had a chronic constipation problem; and I had to take Metamucil every day. Now, I don't have to take it, except occasionally. I have much more energy, and I really feel like a different person. Several of my friends have remarked that my skin looked so much better.

Thank you **so** much for all your help.

Dear Dr. Tessler,

When I first met you, I had been a devout drug addict for twenty-eight years. Cocaine, marijuana, alcohol and nicotine habits had firmly embedded themselves in my system. My coffee intake exceeded six cups a day and was accompanmied by a liberal intake of sugar and heavily salted meals.

As I discovered through your tests, I had been blessed with a strong constitution, which enabled me to survive my highly toxic intake, and I prided myself in a daily exercise regime which allowed me to "look" good at age forty-two. But the blood and hair analysis tests showed me the real truth; the accumulated damage of these excessive and dangerous habits had manifested itself in the functional impairment of most of my organs, and I was about to pay a severe price in the form of one or more disabling diseases. Lung cancer, emphysema, colon cancer, diabetes, arterioschlerosis (from my heavy intake of meat substances) and stroke were distinct near term possibilities. A medical doctor's examination had already indicated a pre-cancerous condition in my lungs, so I knew your assessments were at least credible.

Over a three month period you taught me how to apply the principles of nutrition in my every day life. You advised significant modifications to my diet and vitamin and mineral supplements to feed and support my starving tissues. As I wanted to live without falling prey to the illnesses it was certain I would shortly experience, I followed the program religiously and as I write this testimony, three years later, I have become a healthy human being free of the addictions that plagued me all my adult life. Applying the principles taught to me, I now look forward to a long, healthy vibrant and productive future.

Dear Dr. Tessler,

You have enabled me to find the resources within my own body for fighting pain. The road was not the "instant" cure that most of us want when faced with illness or disease. The methods involved were a change of diet, vitamin therapy and exercise. I thank God that I was guided by you. Without your aid, I would have had unnecessary surgery, many pain killers and a constant fear that "death was at my doorstep."

There were various signs that something was awry with my body before Christmas, 1982. I had begun to have daily headaches which lasted for, at least, eight hours. Their intensity and duration increased.

Now the problem was exacerbated with difficulties in gross and fine motor coordination on the right side of my body. Writing a check at the grocery store became a very difficult experience and I was having great difficulty in climbing stairs.

Once again the problem was compounded with daily afternoon nausea from the headache pain.

Having found no relief from my gynecologist, internist, ophthalmologist, neurologist, and psychiatrist, I now proceeded to search out a good nutritionist.

I went to your free lecture, and immediately scheduled an appointment for hair analysis, blood work, and urine tests. You did not ask me one question concering my symptoms. as every doctor before you had done. You said that the results would show what symptoms I had been experiencing.

I found out that I had copper poisoning, a vitamin B deficiency, and a calcium and magnesium level that was way too low. You explained that I was probably experiencing muscular weakness and that difficulty with writing and walking would be something that I should be experiencing. My severely high copper levels would be given me headaches plus a high white blood count.

Please tell anyone that health does not happen overnight. I struggled for two months before I saw a change. At first, the new diet and supplements actually made me feel worse. I felt weak and tired. But then something did happen. My headaches dropped to four a week, and after a year are virtually non-existent. The color of my skin improved (as the toxins exlted from my body). I generally feel that I have tremendous energy.

For three years I took tetracycline on a regular basis. Well, it has been over one year without tetracycline and no pimples appear **unless** I eat improper foods. And I had always been told by all the dermatologists who I had seen that diet and acne have a very low correlation.

Gordon, I thank you for helping me to find that alternative for a healthy way to live. I appreciate all that you have done for me.

Dear Dr. Tessler,

I wanted to write and let you know how I am doing. As you may recall I had lung problems all my life. As a child it was hay fever, then asthma and then at 13, tuberculosis. I was 16 when I first started having trouble with arthritis.

All my life I had taken so many drugs to breathe that I would get ulcers in my stomach.

If all this wasn't enough, 8 years ago I got an internal parasite that left me with a disease called sprue. My prognosis was that I had about five years to live.

As the sprue got worse, my lungs would fill with fluid and I would get pneumonia. I was always on antibiotics.

When I went to see you I was at the bottom with no hope. As I began your nutritional program, I learned how to eat properly, and what supplements I needed to help my body rebuild itself. Now 3 1/2 years later, I don't have hay fever, asthma, pneumonia, ulcers or arthritis. I am healthier today than ever before in my life.

If someone would have told me 3 1/2 years ago that I could feel this good I would not have believed them (**I AM NOW A BELIEVER**).

Thank you for the knowledge and for all the support you have given me.

Dear Dr. Tessler,

It has taken me some time to get around to this, and since it's almost one year since I first came to you, decided now is the time to write to you and let you know how very greatful and happy I am that I happened to tune into KOA one night about a year and a half ago when I couldn't sleep. It took me six months (and more doctor visits) to determine that something else was necessary. You showed me the way. It wasn't easy, and there were times I felt like stopping - but when I did I was always sorry. I **KNOW** that to keep on feeling top-notch, I must treat my body right.

When I told my husband I had been suffering from malnutrition, he couldn't believe it - since I (we) seemed to have been eating rather well. If only all the people who think the same way could really know what eating right could do for them. I don't feel like a "new person." I feel like the person I used to be and couldn't figure out what had happened to her.

"Old age" was creeping up on me in an insidious way and I didn't like it at all! I now have the energy, the will to do, clearer thinking, and my girlish figure which I thought was gone forever. Everyone who asks me is surprised when I tell them I didn't go on any 'diet' - but it's just a result of eating the right foods - and I certainly have never counted calories or anything of that nature since I started your program. I'm even doing things that I had never done - I might mow the lawn (one or two strips and I've had it) or try to do yard work and get easily fatigued. Now I mow the whole lawn (a rather large one) and work for hours at a time in the yard - as well as handling my husband's office work, taking care of a larger home than previously, and being a bowling secretary. And once again, I'm able to think clearly—and make decisions which had become oh, so hard for me to make.

I also know that now that my body is on the mend - no more headaches, high blood pressure - that if I slip once in awhile, it won't hurt as long as I stay 95% of the time with the right foods. I'm much more active, getting more exercise (walking and biking), sleeping better for the most part and the poor muscle coordination has certainly improved, and I believe the arthritis is also starting to improve.

Thank God for you and your program, and for my husband who gave me moral support when I weakened - although he did say I showed extreme strength in staying with it. And I'm glad I did. Thanks again.

Dear Dr. Tessler,

Thank you . . . . .

_____

Your name

Gordon S. Tessler, Ph.D.
3389 Calle Cancuna
Carlsbad, CA 92009

READING LIST

Dr. Airola's Books - Health Plus Publishing, P.O. Box 22001, Phoenix, Arizona 85028
1. Every Woman's Book
2. How To Get Well
3. Are You Confused?
4. Garlic
5. How To Keep Slim, Healthy & Young Through Juice Fasting
6. Rejuvenation Secrets From Around The World
7. Hypoglycemia - A Better Approach

THE HOLY BIBLE
1. Genesis 1:29
2. Leviticus 11
3. Deuteronomy 14
4. Daniel 1:8-16

VIDEOS

Fit For You, Rebounder Exercise Videos, Sylvia Ortiz, 10820 Beverly Blvd, Suite 308, Whittier, CA 90601, 1-800-521-JUMP

EXERCISE

Fit or Fat - Covert Bailey, Boston, MA

Stretching - Bob Anderson, Shelter Publications, P.O. Box 279, Bolians, CA 94924

COOK BOOKS

The Book of Whole Grains, Marlene Anne Bumgarner, St. Martin's Press, New York

Ten Talents, Frank Hurd, D.C. and Rosalie Hurd, B.S., Dr. and Mrs. Frank J. Hurd, Box 86A, Route 1, Chisolm, MN 55719

Cooking for Optimum Health, Melissa Thompson, available from Trumpets of Zion Ministries, P.O. Box 99005, Raleigh, NC 27624, 919-990-1135

Diet and Salad Suggestions, Dr. Norman Walker, Norwalk Press Publishers, 2218 East Magnolia, Phoenix, AZ 85034

GENERAL NUTRITION

Sugar Blues, William Duffy

Sunlight Could Save Your Life, Zane R. Kime, M.D.

Nature's Seven Doctors, H.E. Kirschner, M.D., H.C. White Publications, P.O. Box 8014, La Sierra, CA

The Colon Health Handbook, Robert Gray, Rockridge Publishing Company, Oakland, CA

Vegetarian Primer, John Revaud, Fox Publications, Dept. 571, 2640 East Twelfth Avenue, Denver, CO 80206

The Changing American Diet, Letitia Brewster and Michael F. Jacobson, Ph.D., (Center for Science in the Public Interest) 1755 S. Street, N.W., Washington, D.C. 20009, (202) 332-9110

WATER

The Shocking Truth About Water, Dr. Paul C. Bragg, Health Science

Flouride, The Aging Factor, Dr. John Yiamouyiannis, Health Action Press

Your Water and Your Health, Dr. Allen E. Banik, Pivot Health

GOVERNMENT PUBLICATIONS

Amino Acid Content of Foods, Home Economics Research Report No. 4, U.S. Dept. of Agriculture, 1968.

Composition of Foods, Agricultural Handbook No. 8, Agricultural Research Service, U.S. Dept. of Agriculture, 1963.

Dietary Goals for the United States, Select Committee on Nutrition and Human Needs—U.S. Senate, U.S. Printing Office, 1977.